COMPREHENSIVE REVIEW GUIDE FOR THE
RADIATION THERAPY
EXAMINATION

LAURA NAPPI B.S. R.T. (R)(T)(M)
RADIATION THERAPIST
INSTRUCTOR

Comprehensive Review Guide For The Radiation Therapy Examination

Copyright © 2017 by Laura Nappi

Copy Editor: Amy Ciauro Stellabotte

Reviewers and Contributors

Daniel Brancato M.S., RTT
Radiation Oncology Manager
The Valley Hosptital

Carol Chovanec M.S., RTT
Program Director
Bergen Community College

Julie Lo M.S. dABR
Physicist
The Valley Hospital

Dr. Thomas Kole M.D., Ph.D.
Radiation Oncologist
The Valley Hospital

Preface

I started to create this study guide for myself when I was a student and subsequently earned a 95 on my Registry exam. Since then, I knew that this would be helpful to others. Therefore, I have worked to constantly improve the material. My goal throughout has been to provide students with the specific information they need to pass their registry exam and help them be prepared for their careers as well.

This review guide follows along with the ARRT content specifications. Therefore, it will help you to study exactly what is necessary to pass the registry. Towards the end of the guide you will find helpful math equations I used to prepare for my exam. At the end of this book you will find two mock registry exams followed by the answer keys. These questions are based on the content found in this book.

I hope this review guide helps you just as much as it helped me. Good luck!
- Laura Nappi

Disclaimers

As a disclaimer, I do not claim the following information as my own original work. I have created a study guide in my own words based on facts that were already created. Use this guide as a supplemental study tool to review for your exam. What I have written is what I believe is important for the exam. For more in depth descriptions refer to the sources I cited at the end of the book. In addition, this field is constantly evolving and changing and therefore ideas and practices may change over time.

The study guide does follow the outline of the ARRT content specifications. However, the ARRT does not review, evaluate, or endorse publications or other educational materials. Permission to reproduce ARRT copyrighted materials should not be construed as an endorsement of the publication by the ARRT.

Table of Contents

Chapter 1: Patient Care

Objectives
- Identify key concepts of patient care
- Define legal terminology
- Understand different ways to communicate
- Understand the importance of communication
- Learn proper techniques for patient transfers
- Identify different types of medical emergencies
- Describe the cycle of infection and infection control
- Discuss ways to screen for and diagnose cancer
- Identify key concepts for documentation

Part 1: Patient Rights

A. Ethics

1. Legal Aspects

a. Informed Consent
- Informed consent forms must be signed by the patient and the doctor
  - » A parent, power of attorney, or health care proxy can sign in place of the patient when the patient is unable to sign
- This form gives the doctor permission to perform a procedure on the patient
- It explains the procedure and the risks and benefits of the procedure, as well as provides alternatives to this procedure
- It is required for invasive procedures, sedation, any procedures that put the patient at risk, and procedures that use radiation
- A **written consent** is an official agreement that has been signed on paper or digitally by everyone involved
- **Verbal consent** gives the doctor permission with a verbal message
- A **simple consent** is expressed or implied permission given for the procedure when the patient does not have enough information about the procedure
  - » **Expressed consent:** Patient does not stop the procedure
    - Patient wants the procedure to occur
  - » **Implied consent:** It is implied that the patient would give consent if the patient's condition permitted
    - Consent could be given by another person if the patient is unable to give consent himself/herself
    - Used for emergency situations
- **Inadequate consent**, or ignorant consent, is when the patient was not given enough information to make the appropriate decision

b. Patient Confidentiality
- **Health Insurance Portability and Accountability Act** (HIPAA) of 1996
  - » Created a standard for the confidentiality of patient records
  - » A patient's information can be talked about only by those who are directly involved in the patient's care

c. Patient's Bill of Rights

- The Patient's Bill of Rights outlines the expectations the patient has of the health care facility that they are involved with
- The patient has the legal right to influence the outcome of his or her treatment
- All patient records are to be kept confidential
- The goal of care should be identified for the patient's treatment
- Radiation therapy treatments have a curative or palliative goal
  - » **Curative** or definitive treatments have a goal to eradicate the tumor
  - » **Palliative** treatments have a goal to alleviate the patient's symptoms, such as reducing pain, stopping pelvic bleeding, improving breathing, etc.
    - Palliative treatments do not intend to prolong patient's life
- **Living wills** are legal documents that state the patient's choice for their health care when they become terminally sick
- The **health care proxy** is a power of attorney, or someone the patient has chosen to make health care decisions for the patient when they are unable to
- Directives such as DNR explain whether or not the patient would like to receive resuscitation or CPR

d. Patient Identification

- Patient identification verification is important so that the correct patient receives the correct treatment
- The patient must be identified in two unique ways
- Visual identification occurs when the therapist compares the photo of the patient in the chart to the patient they will be treating
- Patients may also be identified by their wristbands if they are inpatients or identification cards if they are outpatients
- The patient should confirm their name and date of birth

e. Common Definitions

- **Malpractice:** A professional, such as a physician, unintentionally acts wrongfully, which causes injury to the patient
- **Tort:** Wrongful acts that are intentional or unintentional
- **Battery:** Harmful, unjustifiable acts to or against another person
  - » Physical touch that is meant to harm someone
  - » Physical touch that is not permitted
- **Assault:** A threat of physical touch or harm
- **Negligence:** The medical professional's failure to act or care for the patient, which leads to the patient's injury
  - » Unintentional tort
- **False imprisonment:** Confinement or restraint of the patient without the appropriate approval
- **Libel:** Written defamation of character
  - » Intentional tort

- **Slander:** Verbal defamation of character
  - » Intentional tort
- **Invasion of privacy:** A patient's private information is shared with those who are not involved in the patient's health care
  - » Violation of HIPAA
- **Respondeat superior:** "Let the master answer"
  - » Employers are liable for the negligent acts of their employees
- **Res ipsa loquitur:** "The thing speaks for itself"
  - » The health care worker involved in the negligent act is liable for himself/herself
  - » The health care worker must be able to explain what happened and prove that negligence did not occur

f. Proper Restraints and Immobilizations
- In the health care setting, some patients who might cause harm to themselves may have to be restrained, meaning they need devices to limit any movement in order to prevent injury to themselves or others
- Restraints must be ordered by the appropriate health care provider, such as a physician, physician assistant, or nurse practitioner
- Immobilization devices are made for radiation therapy patients to help create a reproducible setup
- Immobilization devices restrict the patient's movement with the patient's cooperation

B. Communication
1. Types of Communication
a. Verbal
- Verbal communication involves speaking
  - » Example: A doctor is speaking to the radiation therapist about how he or she would like the patient to be set up for treatment

b. Written
- Written communication is recorded information that can be read by others
  - » Example: Test results are sent to the patient via mail with the results typed and printed in a letter

c. Nonverbal
- Nonverbal communication is unspoken
- Examples: nodding, hand gestures, smiling, facial expressions, eye contact, touch, etc.

2. Communication Complications
   a. *Complications In Communicating With Others*
      - Communication may differ with different cultural beliefs, values, and practices
      - Nonverbal and verbal communication may vary in different cultures and societies
      - Symbols and humor may also be different among different cultures
      - Elder patients may be hard of hearing
        » It is important to speak loudly and clearly
      - Elder patients may have memory loss or dementia
        » In this case it is important for a family member to be present with the patient
        » The therapist or other health care worker should speak to the patient and family member
      - Younger children should be spoken to on their level
        » The therapist should kneel or sit next to the patient to be closer to the child's level
      - Adolescents are trying to build their self-esteem, and the therapist must be aware of this
        » The therapist should maintain the adolescent's privacy as much as they can
      - The emotional status of a patient may impair their communication skills temporarily
      - Stages of grieving defined by Elisabeth Kübler-Ross (in order):
        » Denial, anger, bargaining, depression, and acceptance
      - Medical terms and procedures should be explained to the patient in layman's terms

3. Educating the Patient
   a. *Treatment Education*
      - Patients are very nervous on their first day because they do not know what to expect
      - Prior to the patient's treatment, the radiation therapist should explain the procedure to the patient
      - The therapist should take the time to sit down with the patient and explain each step so the patient knows what to expect in the treatment room
      - If the patient has any questions, they should be answered before the procedure starts
      - It is optimal for the patient to be compliant with all procedures that will occur, including tattoo marks and positioning devices
        » Clear explanations of all devices and marks will lead to more patient compliance
        » If the patient understands why the procedure must occur, they will be more compliant
        » If the patient refuses any procedures like tattoo markings, other steps must be taken in order to get a reproducible setup

4. Ancillary Services
   - Support services are available to oncology patients to provide further information as needed
   - Hospice is care for terminally ill patients and focuses on the patient's comfort rather than cure toward the end of his or her life
   - The clergy are religious leaders who provide religious services
   - Social services provide counseling and information to the patient and their families so they can understand and cope with the illness
   - The registered dietitian can help cancer patients manage symptoms caused by radiation therapy or chemotherapy treatments and help maintain a healthy nutritional status

C. Physical Movements

1. Patient Transfer

   a. *Proper Body Mechanics*
   - The lifter should stand with feet separated for a wide base and one foot should be in front of the other
   - The lifter should keep the weight of what they are lifting close to themselves
   - When bending, use knees and hips, not the waist
     » Use muscles in the legs instead of the back
   - Avoid twisting and bending sideways when holding weight

   b. *Transferring Patient's From Wheelchairs and Stretchers*
   - **Wheelchair transfers:** Place wheelchair parallel to table with the wheels locked and footrests out of the way
     » Keep patient's feet together
     » Lifter should face the patient and place their feet on either side of the patient's feet
     » The patient should hold onto the lifter's shoulders while the lifter holds the patient under their arms
       - The patient must not hold the lifter's neck
     » The lifter bends at the knees and hips while lifting the patient and turning the patient until they are seated on the treatment table
     » If the patient needs assistance lying down, place one arm under the patient's shoulders and the other under the knees and turn the patient until they are supine
   - **Stretcher transfers:** Two or more lifters should transfer the patient
     » Place the stretcher at the same height as the treatment table and lower the side rails on the stretcher
     » Use a sheet and sliding board to reduce risk of injury to the lifters
       - Roll the patient away and place the board underneath the sheet under the patient
       - Roll the patient back so their back is on the board
       - Pull the board and patient to the treatment table
       - Remove the board so it is not in the way of the radiation beam
     » When rolling the patient is not ideal, the patient can be moved with more lifters
       - Lifters should be positioned to support the patient's head, hips, shoulders, and feet
       - The patient is lifted with a sheet and moved over to the treatment table
       - Communicate with lifters so everyone lifts the patient at the same time

   c. *Fall Risks*
   - When walking a patient into the treatment room, it is important to walk close to them just in case they lose their balance or trip
   - If a patient requires a wheelchair for assistance, make sure to use one to prevent a fall
   - When the patient is on the patient support assembly (PSA), safety straps may be used to keep the patient in place and to prevent a fall

2. Patients With Medical Devices
   a. *Intravenous Fluids*
   - During the transfer of a patients with an IV placed in the arm, support the arm so the IV is not accidentally displaced
   - The bag of fluid entering the IV should be placed 18" to 24" above the vein

   b. *Oxygen*
   - Oxygen is delivered through outlets in the walls of the hospital or treatment room, or through an oxygen tank
   - The amount of oxygen and the device used to deliver the oxygen is determined by the patient's physician
   - When transferring a patient with oxygen and switching the oxygen from the patient's tank to the treatment room's oxygen connection, be sure to select the correct and prescribed setting for the oxygen flow rate

   c. *Urinary Catheters and Chest Tubes*
   - If a patient has a urinary catheter, ensure that urine drainage bags are placed below the level of the bladder so urine does not flow back into the bladder
     » Never empty the drainage bag, because the patient's urinary output is measured and recorded
   - If the patient has chest tubes, the tubes should always be kept straight and unclamped
     » Should be kept below the level of the patient's chest

D. Patients With Medical Emergencies
1. Drug Allergies
   - Allergic reactions are negative reactions to drugs
   - When the drug enters the patient, the body thinks of the drug as an antigen and creates antibodies for that drug
   - The more the patient is exposed to the drug they are allergic to, the more sensitive the patient becomes and reactions could become more severe
   - **Minor** reactions to contrast media are nausea, hives, mild vomiting, weakness, warmth, pallor, etc.
     » Patient doesn't need to seek medical treatment, but must be observed to ensure reaction does not get worse
   - **Moderate** reactions to contrast media are tachycardia, bradycardia, hypotension, hypertension, dyspnea, laryngeal edema, etc.
     » Patient doesn't need to seek medical treatment, but must be observed to ensure reaction does not get worse
   - A **severe** reaction to contrast media or drugs is anaphylactic shock
     » During an anaphylactic shock, the patient experiences respiratory arrest and vascular shock
     » Some common symptoms are laryngeal edema, convulsions, unresponsiveness, extreme hypotension, nausea, etc.
     » Epinephrine can be used as a treatment

» Treatment must occur rapidly

- Contraindications for using contrast media are patients older than the age of 50, patients with diabetes, patients with limited kidney function, patients with heart disease, or patients who have had previous adverse reactions to contrast media

2. Cardiopulmonary Resuscitation

- Cardiopulmonary resuscitation (CPR) is needed when the patient goes into cardiac arrest
- Begin CPR if a patient's pulse stops
- The proper steps taken to assess the patient prior to starting CPR are C-A-B (circulation, airway, breathing)
- To correctly perform CPR, perform chest compressions if the patient has no pulse, check the airway and open up the airway up by tilting the patient's head, and perform mouth-to-mouth breathing techniques
- The ratio of compressions to breaths for an adult is 30:2

3. Injuries and Traumas

- Immediately call for the doctor after an injury occurs
- Then continue to attend to the patient
- Carefully help the patient without causing further injury
- After the incident has occurred, an incident report may need to be filled out according to the facility's rules

4. Seizures and Diabetes

- **Seizures:**
  - » When a patient has a seizure, it is important to stay with them
  - » Monitor the patient so they do not cause any injuries
  - » Call for help and assistance
  - » Do not put your fingers into the patient's mouth and do not restrain the patient
- **Diabetic Reactions:**
  - » Hypoglycemia is when there is too much insulin
    - Caused when the patient hasn't had anything to eat or drink
  - » Diabetic ketoacidosis is when there isn't enough insulin
    - Treatment is IV and/or insulin
  - » When these reactions occur, stop all procedures and remain with the patient
  - » Call an emergency team and monitor the patient's vital signs
  - » Can be deadly if untreated

E. Infection Control and Prevention

1. Sequence of Infection

   a. Pathogen
   - A microorganism that causes an infectious disease

   b. Source of Infection
   - Infectious microorganisms originate from a source
   - The infectious microorganisms are then transferred through a host via direct or indirect contact
   - Infectious microorganisms have the ability to live and duplicate within the reservoir

   c. Portal of Entry or Exit
   - The host of the infectious microorganism must have a portal of entry or exit in order for the disease to be spread
     » Examples: blood, skin, respiratory tract, gastrointestinal tract

   d. Ways of Transmission
   - Direct
     » **Direct contact:** The host physically touches the source of infection
       - Examples: touch, kiss, sexual intercourse
       - The most common method of transmission
     » **Droplet:** The source of infection is transferred through air quickly, in large particles, and in short distances
       - Examples: talking, coughing, sneezing
       - Mumps, rubella, influenza, and pneumonia can be transmitted though droplets
   - Indirect
     » The host touches an object that has been infected by the source of infection
       - Example: needles
     » Herpes, impetigo, scabies, and zoster can be transmitted through indirect contact
     » **Airborne:** The source of infection is transmitted through long distances in air and in small particles
       - Particles can stay in the air for hours to days
       - Examples: measles, varicella, and tuberculosis
     » **Vehicle-borne:** Many people can become infected when in contact with a contaminated fomite
       - Fomites are inanimate objects like food, water, medications, and equipment
       - Can contaminate multiple people
     » **Vector-borne:** An infectious vector transports the microorganisms
       - Examples: flies, mosquitos, ticks, and rats

   e. Host
   - The host is where the infectious microorganism is passed
   - The host needs to have a portal of entry
     » Examples: skin, mouth, etc.

2. Methods of Disinfection and Sterilization
   a. *Disinfection*
   - Disinfection decreases the number of microorganisms
   - Boiling water and chemical liquids can disinfect equipment
   - There are various types of chemical disinfectants that can be effective for different types of infectious agents
     » Examples: germicides, bactericides, fungicides, and virucides

   b. *Sterilization*
   - Sterilization completely destroys all organisms and spores
   - Moist or dry heat, steam under pressure, chemical sterilization, and ethylene oxide can sterilize equipment
   - Steam sterilizers are also known as steam autoclaves
     » Most common way to sterilize equipment

   c. *Medical Asepsis*
   - Medical asepsis decreases the amount of microorganisms
   - Unlike sterile technique, medical asepsis does not completely remove spores

3. Standard Precautions
   a. *Hand Washing*
   - The number one way to reduce nosocomial infections is proper hand hygiene
   - Hands must be washed after touching blood, other body fluids, and other secretions or excretions
   - After gloves are removed, hands should be washed
   - Hands should always be washed between treating patients

   b. *Gloves, Gowns, and Masks*
   - Gloves should be worn when touching blood, body fluids, contaminated articles, mucous membranes, and skin that is not intact
   - Gloves must be changed between procedures on the same patient
   - A gown is worn to protect skin and clothing
   - A mask should be worn when a procedure is likely to cause splashes or sprays of blood or other body fluids
   - Particulate respirators protect the worker against small droplet nuclei

   c. *Needles*
   - Never recap needles after use to avoid needle sticks
   - If needle stick occurs, it must be reported immediately
   - Discard in labeled, puncture-resistant containers after use
     » Containers should be kept close to the area where needles are being used
   - Never use the same needle for different patients
   - Do not bend or break needles with hands

d. Handling and Disposal of Contaminated Material
- Always handle very carefully to keep the contamination from spreading to other materials
- Contaminated equipment that is a single-use piece of equipment must be discarded properly
- Contaminated equipment that can be reused must be cleaned or sterilized before being used again
- Linens that have been contaminated must be handled with gloves and placed in a labeled biohazard bag that won't leak
- Contaminated linens are thrown away or placed in a labeled bag to be sent for decontamination
- Other linens used daily must be placed in a bin located in the treatment room so that they can be cleaned before reuse
- Linens should be changed before treating each patient
- Sharp equipment that can be disposed of, such as needles, must be placed in a puncture-resistant container
- Supplies should be used for only one patient
- Used supplies should be sent to be re-sterilized or should be thrown away
- Alpha-cradles cannot be reused and must be thrown away
- Vac-locks can be reused but must be properly cleaned between patients
- Patient blood and body fluid leaks should be cleaned up immediately
  » Use proper disinfectants or a bleach solution

4. Transmission-Based Precautions
  a. Contact Precautions
- Wear gloves while in the room and wear a gown if in contact with the patient or their linen
- Wash hands before going into the patient's room and when leaving the patient's room
- Wash hands if handling the patient's body fluids

  b. Droplet Precautions
- A surgical mask must be worn in and near the patient's room
- Wash hands before going into the patient's room and when leaving the patient's room
- Wash hands if handling the patient's body fluids

  c. Airborne Precautions
- HEPA filter or negative air-pressure room is used for patients with tuberculosis
- Wash hands before going into the patient's room and when leaving the patient's room
- Wash hands if handling the patient's body fluids
- N95 or HEPA respirator masks for workers
- Standard masks for visitors

5. Other Precautions
   a. *Reverse Isolation*
   - Reverse isolation is used for immunosuppressed patients
   - Protects the patient from any infectious microorganisms the staff or visitors may have
   - Those entering the patient's room must wear a mask, a gown, and gloves

   b. *Nosocomial Infections*
   - Nosocomial infections are acquired within the health care setting
   - These infections can be caused from environmental aspects of the facility
     » Examples: airflow, temperature, humidity, carpeting, furniture, plants, etc.

F. Handling and Disposal of Dangerous Materials
1. Materials
   a. *Metals*
   - Shielding blocks are made of bismuth, lead, tin, and cadmium
     » Lipowitz metal or Cerrobend
   - The most toxic materials are lead and cadmium
     » Cadmium dust can affect the lungs and kidneys
     » Lead can affect the brain
   - Toxicities may transpire if the materials are breathed in or absorbed through the skin, or if someone eats or drinks contaminated foods
   - When handling blocks or cutouts, protective clothing, eyewear, and gloves must be worn
   - Workers must wash their hands after touching the blocks or cutouts
   - The melting pot should be kept below a fume hood to properly filter the toxic fumes from the air
   - There are more toxic fumes as the temperature of the melting pot increases
   - The temperature of the melting pot should not be any higher than 85°C
   - Standards for handling of and exposure to toxic materials are set by OSHA

   b. *Chemicals*
   - Chemicals are examples of carcinogens
   - DNA can be mutated as a reaction to chemicals
   - Protective gear should be worn when handling chemicals

   c. *Radioactive Materials*
   - Must abide by ALARA (time, distance, and shielding) when around radioactive materials to keep exposure to a minimum
     » ALARA stands for As Low As Reasonably Achievable
   - Must wear proper personal protection when handling radioactive materials
   - Eating and drinking in areas where radioactive materials are being handled is not allowed

d. Chemotherapy
- When preparing and administering chemotherapy, personnel must wear gloves, gowns, and face shields
- If spilled on the skin, some chemotherapy drugs may cause blisters or ulcers
- After a spill of liquid chemotherapy, a towel or a spill kit is used to clean up and is then disposed of in a biohazard bag
    » The area must be cleaned with detergent

2. Material Safety Data Sheet (MSDS)
- Data sheets that give information about how to use and handle specific chemicals and materials in a safe way
- Provides information about the chemical's physical property, like the melting point of the material
- Provides information about the health effects that can be caused by materials
- Provides information about the reactivity of the chemicals
- Provides information on how to store and dispose of the materials

Part 2: Patient Charts and Records

A. Evaluating Diseases

1. Etiology
   - Etiology is the study of what causes the disease
   - There is no known specific cause of cancer
   - Examples of etiology factors include cigarette smoke, human papillomavirus (HPV), alcohol, genetics, and sun exposure

2. Epidemiology
   - Epidemiology is the study how many people have a disease
   - The frequency of disease is affected by factors such as age, gender, race, occupation, and geographic location

3. Screening Tests
   - Screening tests can detect cancer before a patient will show any symptoms
   - Tests must be sensitive and specific
     » **Sensitive** means it can accurately detect a tumor in the early stages
     » **Specific** means it can detect a particular type of cancer
   - Not all types of cancer have screening tests
   - The Pap smear (Papanicolau smear) screens for cervical cancer
     » Recommended to have Pap smears routinely after age 21
   - Fecal occult blood tests or a colonoscopy screens for colorectal cancer
     » Recommended to have colonoscopies routinely after age 50
   - Mammograms screen for breast cancer
     » Recommended to have mammograms annually after age 40
   - Digital rectal exam and prostate-specific antigen (PSA) are screening tests for prostate cancer
     » Recommended to have tests after age 50

4. Signs and Symptoms of Disease
   - A **sign** is an indication of disease observed by someone who is examining the patient (objective)
     » Example: the doctor sees a change in the patient's mole
   - A **symptom** is an indication of disease that is observed by the patient (subjective)
     » Example: the patient feels pain or nausea

5. Physical Examination
- Patients can provide information on their history of health and their family history of health
- Vital signs: temperature, pulse, respirations, and blood pressure
  - » Normal temperature = 97 to 99 degrees
    - Temperature can be taken at the mouth, axilla and rectum
  - » Normal pulse for an adult = 70 to 100 beats per minute
    - Radial artery is the most common location to measure pulse
    - Apical artery is the most accurate location to measure pulse
  - » Normal adult respiration rate = 14 to 16 breaths per minute
  - » Normal adult blood pressure = 90 to 140 mm Hg (systolic) and 60 to 90 mm Hg (diastolic)

6. Diagnostic Imaging
- **Nuclear medicine (PET scans):** injects a radioactive material into a patient that releases gamma rays and then the uptake can be imaged and the radiation is measured
  - » Shows the body's anatomy and function
- **Radiographs:** 2-D images of the body such as chest x-ray, abdomen (KUB), etc.
- **Computed tomography (CT):** 3-D images of the body that show more detail than radiographs and can visualize the contrast of air, soft tissue and bone
- **Magnetic resonance imaging (MRI):** 3-D images that use radiofrequency waves and a magnetic field
  - » Doesn't use radiation
  - » Shows soft tissue better than CT or radiographs
- **Diagnostic ultrasound:** uses high-frequency sound waves to image soft tissue within the body

7. Diagnostic Studies
  a. Lab
- Blood work examines blood, bone marrow, urine, feces, etc.
- Detects tumor markers
- Normal ranges in complete blood count as stated by the Mayo Clinic:

White blood cells	3.50 –10.5 billion cells/L
Red blood cells	3.90 – 5.70 million/mcL
Hemoglobin	12.0 – 17.5 g/dL
Hematocrit	34.9 – 50.0%
Platelets	150,000 – 450,000/mcL

  b. Surgical Biopsies
- The diagnosis of cancer can be confirmed only with a biopsy
  - » **Incisional biopsy:** removal of a segment of the tumor
  - » **Excisional biopsy:** removal of the whole tumor
- The report also states what part of the body was biopsied and any lymph nodes that were tested as well

c. Pathology
- The pathology report states the histopathologic diagnosis of the removed tissue
- Gives specific diagnosis of the cell type

B. Patient Evaluation
1. Side Effects From Radiation Treatments
a. Signs and Symptoms
- Patients are observed throughout the course of their treatment
- Patients have weekly visits with the doctor so the doctor can evaluate any signs that may appear as a result of radiation therapy
- On a daily basis, if a patient feels any symptoms, they should tell the radiation therapist or nurse prior to treatment
  - » Sometimes it may be necessary to have a break in treatments in order for the patient to heal more before continuing

b. Radiation Related Side Effects
- Radiation can cause different side effects when treating different parts of the body
- The extent of the side effect varies with dose
- Chemotherapy can cause side effects such as mucositis, stomatitis, esophagitis, epilation, pneumonitis, myelopathy, etc.
- The following chart shows side effects and the doses they occur

Faint erythema	1,600 cGy
Erythema	2,000 cGy
Dry desquamation	3,000 cGy
Moist desquamation	4,000 cGy
Epilation	Temporary: 2,000 cGy or Permanent: 4,500 cGy
Stomatitis, xerostomia, mucositis, taste alterations	2,000 cGy
Pharyngitis	2,000 – 3,000 cGy
Laryngitis	4,000 cGy
Esophagitis	2,000 – 3,000 cGy
Nausea/vomiting	1,000 – 3,000 cGy
Diarrhea	2,000 cGy
Cystitis	3,000 cGy
Cataracts	Total of 1,000 cGy or single treatment of 200 cGy
Sterility of testes	Temporary: <500 or Permanent: >500 cGy
Bone and soft-tissue necrosis	6,000 cGy

c. Management
- Skin reactions to radiation should be observed for any changes or open sores
  - » Moisturizing lotions should be used as prescribed
  - » Lotions with alcohol or scents should be avoided
  - » The patient should wear loose clothing and clothes made with cotton
  - » The area should be well ventilated
  - » Avoid heat, cold, soaps, deodorants, razor shaving, and direct sunlight

»   If there is skin breakdown, the oncologist might temporarily stop the patient's treatments so the skin has time to heal

- When the patient is dealing with radiation side effects of the mouth and stomach, a soft, bland diet may be implemented
- For pharyngitis, laryngitis, and esophagitis, the patient should only eat room-temperature, soft, non-spicy, and nonacidic foods
  »   Topical anesthetics and analgesics may be prescribed
- Nausea and vomiting must be managed with fluids to avoid dehydration
  »   Patient should be put on a low-fat and low-sugar diet
- If the patient has diarrhea, they should be put on a low-residue diet
  »   Antispasmodic medications can be prescribed if needed
- Antiemetic (treats nausea) medications are Torecan, Norazine, and Compazine
- Analgesic (pain killer) medications are Tylenol, Percocet, and MS Contin
- Anti-inflammatory medications are hydrocortisone and Diprolene
- Antidiarrheal medications are Imodium and Lomotil

2. Blood Work
  a. Different Types of Blood Studies
  - **CBC** (complete blood count): assesses the amount of red blood cells, white blood cells, hemoglobin (oxygen-carrying protein), hematocrit (proportion of RBCs to the fluid/plasma), and platelets
  - **BUN** (blood urea nitrogen): blood test that evaluates kidney and liver function
  - **Creatinine:** measures the amount of creatinine in the blood, which evaluates the kidney function
    »   If there are high levels of creatinine, this means the kidneys are not filtering properly

  b. Reasons For Changes In Blood Work
  - Blood counts may be altered by other health issues or if the kidneys and/or liver are not functioning properly
  - Chemotherapy and radiation therapy can affect blood values
  - Chemotherapy such as MOPP causes myelosuppression, which is a decrease in white blood cells, red blood cells, and platelets
  - Bone marrow depression occurs when more than 25 percent of bone marrow is within the radiation treatment field
    »   Most bone marrow is located in the pelvis
    »   Bone marrow is also commonly located in the vertebrae and long bones of the extremities

3. Dietary Intervention
  a. Common Dietary Related Issues
  - Weight loss is a common problem with patients receiving radiation therapy
  - Weight loss signifies tissue loss
  - **Anorexia:** the loss of appetite that leads to weight loss
    »   Leads to cancer cachexia

- **Cachexia:** malnutrition and wasting due to an illness
  - » Early satiety, electrolyte imbalance and water imbalance disease
  - » Loss of fat and muscle
- Radiation therapy and chemotherapy can cause certain digestive issues
- Patients getting radiation therapy treatments to their head, neck, or chest can experience a sore throat
  - » If the treatment is specifically in the mouth, the patient may experience soreness within the mouth, which will cause difficulty chewing and swallowing
  - » Sore and irritated mouth or throat can lead to difficulties with eating and therefore lead to weight loss
  - » Treatments to the thorax can cause esophagitis and dsyphagia
- This can be noticed within the first three weeks of treatment
- Patients getting radiation therapy to the abdominal region may experience diarrhea, nausea, and/or vomiting
  - » Diarrhea can cause poor appetite, dehydration, weakness, and/or weight loss
- Dietary related side effects differ depending on radiation dose, treatment site, and use of chemotherapy

b. Managing Dietary Related Issues
- Nurses and nutrition specialists should evaluate the patient's nutritional status
  - » Baseline data should be obtained on the first physical examination so the patient can be monitored for changes throughout the treatment
- Patients should receive dietary education from a specialist early on in their treatment in order to prevent or minimize any effects
  - » High-calorie and high-protein diets are encouraged
- Radiation therapists should refer the patient to a nurse or nutritional specialist if changes in weight are noticed
  - » Especially if the patient loses 5% of their body weight in one month or 10% of their body weight in six months
  - » The patient's weight should be checked weekly
- Hyperalimentation: nutrients given through IV for patients who are weak and malnourished
- Patients receiving radiation treatment to the head are likely to experience difficulty swallowing and it can become difficult to receive proper nutrition
  - » Some patients may need a PEG (percutaneous endoscopic gastrostomy) tube
  - » If the patient did not get a PEG tube they may need a prescription for an anesthetic mouth rinse in order to tolerate eating meals
  - » These patients may also experience a change in taste and saliva levels
  - » It can take six months or longer for these patient's to notice improvements in their taste
- To manage a sore mouth, the patient should eat soft, bland foods that are cold or at room temperature
- To manage a sore throat, the patient should eat soft, bland foods that are semi-solid and easy to swallow
  - » Eating smaller, more frequent meals may help the patient avoid discomfort
- To manage nausea, the patient should eat several small meals (foods should be bland and

dry) and drink beverages that have calories and nutrients and provide hydration
- To manage diarrhea, the patient should drink fluids and eat foods with sodium and potassium, as well as avoid eating foods that are high in fiber
- In addition to these precautions, nausea, vomiting, and diarrhea caused by radiation therapy may require prescription medications in order to be managed best

4. On Treatment Visits
- Prior to the start of radiation treatments patients have a physical exam and are evaluated on their height, weight, body mass index (BMI), muscle tone, skin, appearance, and performance status (based on Karnofsky performance status)
- Patients are typically monitored by a nurse and doctor once per week
- During these treatment visits, the patient's weight and vital signs are taken
- The patient is also assessed for any signs or symptoms that may be a result of the radiation therapy treatment
  » They are examined for things like skin erythema, pain, esophagitis, etc.
  » They are asked if they are feeling tired, weak, nauseated, etc.
- All information is documented in the patient's chart

C. Documenting in Patient Charts
1. Important Information
a. Prescription
- Part of the patient's chart includes the prescription for the course of their treatment
- The prescription is written by the radiation oncologist
- The prescription will include the type of radiation, the beam energy, the dose per fraction, the total dose, the amount of fractions, bolus, gating, imaging, etc.
  » Examples: photons or electrons
  » Examples: 6 MV, 15 MV, 6E, 9E, etc.
  » The prescription could also indicate that mixed energies will be used

b. Monitor Units or Time
- Linear accelerators are "on" for a specific amount of monitor units
- Cobalt-60 machines are "on" for a specific amount of time or minutes
  » Gamma Knife and HDR units also use time
- The amount of time or monitor units for each patient's treatment is determined during treatment planning
- MU and time should be documented in the patient's chart or treatment plan

c. Daily and Accumulated Doses
- Therapists record the daily dose and accumulated dose in the patient's chart along side the date of the treatment and fraction number
- Typically, there are two different columns in the treatment chart
  » One column will list the daily doses
  » Another column will list the accumulated doses
- An example of a curative dose is daily fractions of 180 to 200 cGy to a total dose of 5,400 to 6,000 cGy
- An example of a palliative dose is a daily fraction of 300 cGy to a total dose of 3,000 cGy

d. Time of Day for B.I.D. Treatment
- B.I.D. treatments mean the patient is treated twice in one day
- At least six hours must pass before the second treatment is given
- The time of each fraction must be recorded to ensure six hours have elapsed

e. Fraction and Elapsed Days
- Each fraction number should be recorded along with the date and dose
- Each day from the start of treatment to the end of treatment is recorded as "elapsed days"
  » Some facilities begin recording the first treatment day as "0"
  » Other facilities begin recording the first treatment day as "1"
- Days in between treatments are included in this record as well, such as weekends or breaks

f. Treatment Plan Elements
- The treatment plan will also have information on the type of radiation and energy
- Each field has its own name and field number
  » Example: 1 AP
- The field has a specified gantry angle, collimator angle, etc.
- If the field is changed during the course of a treatment, the new field might have subscript letters or other marks to show a change
  » Example: field 1 AP has a change and is renamed field 1a AP

g. Dose Volume Histogram
- Doses to other organs may be found on the DVH (dose volume histogram)
- Some facilities may record the daily dose to the spinal cord if it is receiving a large amount

h. Patient Setup Instructions
- Information from the simulation should be recorded in order to reproduce the setup for the patient's treatment
- Examples of necessary information: gantry angle, SSD, collimator size, collimator angle, couch angle, MLCs, patient's position, neck rolls, immobilization devices, tattoo locations, bolus, etc.
- The patient's position should describe the patient's orientation, such as "head-first supine" or "feet-first supine," for example
- Photographs in the patient's chart are helpful to show the patient's position

2. Important Components of Patient Records

a. Patient Identification

- Patient's identity must be confirmed in two ways
  - » Example: patient's name and date of birth
- A face photo of the patient should be included in the patient's chart for visual confirmation
- The best way to ID an inpatient is with their wrist bracelet
- An outpatient should carry an identification card that will be checked by therapists treating the patient

b. Documentation

- Entries on the patient's chart must be dated and initialed or signed by the radiation therapists who treated the patient
- Information written in a patient's chart must be clear and legible
- If a correction is made, the original record must remain legible
- If an error is made in the treatment chart, draw a single line through the error and then write the correct information
- Add the initials of who corrected it, along with the date
- Never use correction fluid (Wite-Out) or anything that completely covers the error

c. Treatment Changes

- Sometimes a change in treatment is necessary depending on the patient's circumstances
- It is important the therapist treating the patient is aware of any changes and takes the appropriate measures following any changes
  - » For example, changes in field size will require imaging to validate changes
- If there is a change in the field, it will be renamed to show the change
  - » Examples of changed names can be subscript letters, numbers, or prime marks (',")

d. Medical Events

- According to the NRC, a medical event is when the total dose delivered to a patient is different from the prescription by 20 percent or more
- A medical event is also when the delivered dose for one fraction is different from the prescription by 50 percent or more
- Other examples of medical events are if the radioactive materials were delivered to the wrong patient, the radioactive materials were delivered via the wrong route, the wrong radioactive materials were used, or if there was leakage from the sealed source
- The medical event must be reported to the NRC by the next day after the realization of the medical event
  - » A written report must be submitted within 15 days
  - » The patient and the physician must be informed within 24 hours
- The report must include the licensed person's name, the physician who prescribed the treatment, a description of what occurred, the effect on the patient, and the appropriate measures that will be taken after the event
  - » The Radiation Safety Officer (RSO) is responsible for creating these reports

3. Charge Capture Terminology
  a. *Professional and Technical Charges*
    - Professional charges are for the patient care procedures that involve the radiation oncologist
    - Technical charges are for other patient care procedures that do not involve the radiation oncologist
      » Physics and treatment charges
      » Patient is billed every treatment

  b. *CPT Principles (Current Procedural Terminology)*
    - Patients are billed for the treatments they get, the devices they use, and their simulations
    - Billing codes can be broken down into three categories
      » Simple, intermediate and complex
    - Simple devices are devices that can be used for multiple patients
      » Examples: prone pillow, Duncan mask, wing board
    - Intermediate devices are devices that can be indexed and have multiple pieces
    - Complex devices are devices that are custom made and can be used for only one patient
      » Examples: Vac-lok, Alpha Cradles, Aquaplast masks
    - Devices that are used for patient comfort do not require a billing charge
      » Examples: pillows and mats
    - Devices are billed to the patient only once
    - Simple simulations are simulations of a single treatment site without any custom blocking
      » When patients come back for their simulation verification, or dry run prior to the start of treatment, this will be billed as a simple simulation
    - Intermediate simulations are simulations for two or more treatment sites
    - Complex simulations are simulations for treatments using arc therapy, complex or custom blocking, or three or more treatment sites
    - Simple treatments are a single treatment area with only one or two treatment fields and fewer than two simple blocks
    - Intermediate treatment fields are two separate treatment areas and can have at least three treatment fields and three simple blocks
    - Complex treatments can be three or more treatment areas and use custom blocks, tangential fields, wedges, arcs, field-in-field, or electron beams
    - All treatment charges listed above are for treatments using more than 1 MeV
    - Patients are also billed a separate charge for their weekly port images
    - If patients are having a complex treatment that requires IGRT (image-guided radiation therapy), they must be billed for that daily as well
    - IMRT (intensity modulated radiation therapy) has its own charge as well
      » IMRT simple is billed for breast and prostate
      » IMRT complex is for all other IMRT cases

Chapter 2: Radiation Safety

Objectives
- Explain the different sources of radiation
- Review basic concepts of radiation
- Identify the different parts of the linear accelerator and CT simulator
- Learn about the different quality assurance procedures
- Review different effects of radiation
- Discuss tolerances of radiation
- Define the units of measurement for radiation
- Define instruments that measure radiation
- Explain methods of radiation protection

Part 1: Radiation Physics

A. Radiation Sources

1. <u>Radioactive Sources</u>
   - Radioactive materials can be used for diagnostic tests like nuclear medicine
     - » Example: Technetium-99m
   - Radioactive materials can be used for therapeutic purposes
     - » Examples: Palladium-103, Iodine-125, Iridium-192, Cobalt-60 and Strontium-90
   - External beam therapy (or teletherapy) uses radioactive materials, such as Cobalt-60, or man-made radiation to produce an external beam of radiation that is aimed at the patient's body in order to treat cancers
   - Brachytherapy is a "short-distance therapy" that uses radioactive materials to treat certain cancers internally
   - Materials used in brachytherapy can be placed near the tumor or directly inside the tumor
   - Radium (Ra-226) was the original radioactive isotope, which helped start brachytherapy
     - » No longer used today due to some potential hazards
   - There are different types of brachytherapy applicators
     - » **Intraluminal** applicators treat tumors in the lung or esophagus using a single catheter
     - » **Intracavitary** applicators treat tumors in the vagina or cervix
       - Examples: vaginal cylinders, tandem and ovoids, and tandem and ring (Fletcher-Suit)
     - » **Interstitial** applicators are needles or an arrangement of catheters that are used to insert permanent implants, such as I-125 seeds into the prostate
   - Radioactive materials for permanent brachytherapy implants must have low energies and short half-lives so that the radiation cannot travel farther than within the patient's body and cause harm to the public
   - Radioactive materials for temporary brachytherapy can have higher energies because the source will be removed from the patient before he or she leaves the treatment room
     - » Treatment rooms must be appropriately shielded
   - The most common radioisotopes used in brachytherapy are considered to be sealed sources, which means they are covered by metal casings
     - » I-131 is an exception and is not a sealed source
   - Sources that are used for low dose rate (LDR) brachytherapy have activities with a range from 0.1 to 100 mCi

- Sources used for high dose rate (HDR) brachytherapy have activities ranging as high as 10 Ci
- The term **activity** is defined as the strength of radioactive source that is determined by the rate of decay
  - » 1 Curie (Ci) = 3.7 x 10^{10} disintegrations per second (dps)
  - » 1 Becquerel (Bq) = 1 dps
  - » Becquerel is the SI unit
- The half-life of a radioactive source describes the duration of time it takes for the activity to decay to half of the original value
- Cobalt-60 has a half-life of 5.26 years, d_{max} of 0.5 cm, and emits gamma rays from the nucleus with two energies
  - » The two energies emitted by Cobalt-60 are 1.17 and 1.33 MeV
  - » Average energy is 1.25 MeV
  - » Output for Cobalt-60 treatment machines decreases by 1.09 percent per month because of decay
  - » To determine penumbra for Cobalt-60 treatment machines, use the following equations: Penumbra = (s(SSD + d – SDD))/SDD
    - s = source size
    - d = depth
    - SSD = source to skin distance
    - SDD = source to diaphragm/collimator distance
- The following sources are commonly used in radiation therapy. The chart explains the half-life and common uses of each source.

Source	Half-Life	Examples of Use
Iodine (I-131)	8 days	Thyroid cancer treatment
Iodine (I-125)	60.2 days	Permanent implants for treatment of brain and prostate cancers Temporary ocular plaques
Palladium (Pd-103)	17 days	Permanent implants for the treatment of prostate cancers
Cesium (C-137)	30 years	LDR treatment of cancers of the cervix
Strontium (Sr-90)	28.8 years	Treats cancers in the eye
Strontium (Sr-89)	50.5 days	Treats pain caused by bone metastasis
Yttrium (Y-90)	2.67 days	Liver cancer and lymphoma treatments
Iridium (Ir-192)	73.8 days	HDR treatments
Gold (Au-198)	2.7 days	Permanent implants for the treatment of prostate cancer
Radium (Ra-226)	1,622 years	Original radioactive isotope
Cobalt (Co-60)	5.26 years	External beam treatments/ teletherapy

2. Man-Made Radiation

- Photon radiation is created in an x-ray tube or in a linear accelerator when a stream of accelerated electrons hit a tungsten target
  - » Tungsten has a high Z number (atomic number)
- Electrons are accelerated to high energies by high-frequency electromagnetic waves
- Produced in kilovoltage for diagnostic x-ray machines
- Produced in megavoltage for linear accelerators for radiation therapy
- In diagnostic x-ray tubes, electrons are released by the cathode (negative electrode) and are accelerated across a vacuumed tube toward the target on the rotating anode (positive electrode)
  - » There is a potential difference, also known as tube voltage, within the tube
  - » Voltage is supplied by a generator
- Therapy tubes use a similar concept for x-ray production, however, a hooded anode is used instead of a rotating anode
  - » Hooded anodes prevent unwanted secondary electrons
- Targets in therapy machines are known as transmission targets
- Therapy x-ray photons have energies from 50 keV to 25 MeV
- Common beam energies for linear accelerators range from 4MV to 25MV
- Orthovoltage energies range from 150 to 500 kV
- Superficial therapy energies range from 50 to 150 kV
- A cyclotron is used in proton therapy
  - » Cyclotrons speed up the protons
  - » The proton speed determines the energy
  - » High-energy protons are more penetrating than low-energy protons

B. Physics of Radiation

1. Properties of a Wave

- There are three physical characteristics of a wave: frequency, wavelength, and velocity
  - » **Frequency:** the number of waves that pass through a point in a certain amount of time
  - » **Wavelength:** the measured distance between two specific points of the wave (peak to peak, valley to valley, etc.)
    - Measured in meters
    - As the wavelength decreases, the energy increases (inverse relationship)
  - » **Speed:** how fast the wave is traveling
    - Travels at the speed of light (3×10^8 m/sec) in a vacuum
- Photons have both wave and particle characteristics
- Photons have no mass or charge and low LET (linear energy transfer)

2. Attenuation of Matter

- As the radiation beam travels through matter, it will diverge and decrease in intensity by the inverse-square effect
- The beam decreases in intensity because it is either absorbed or scattered in a different direction as it travels through matter
- The beam's intensity will decrease more as the thickness of attenuating material increases

- Determined by the following equation:
    » $I(x) = I_0 e^{-ux}$
        - I_0 = initial intensity
        - u = linear attenuation coefficient (changes depending on composition of the material and beam energy)
        - x = thickness of absorption material
        - Equation applies to monoenergetic beams

3. Inverse-Square Law
    - The radiation beam intensity will decrease with increasing distance due to the beam's divergence
    - Intensity = $1/(d^2)$
        » d = distance
        » Beam intensity is inversely proportional to square of distance from source
    - $I_2/I_1 = (D_1/D_2)^2$
        » I = intensity
        » D = distance
    - Example: if distance increases by two, then intensity decreases by four
    - Example: if distance decreases by two, then intensity increases by four
    - Percentage depth dose equations use the inverse-square law when implementing the "Mayneord F" factor

4. Radiation Beam Quality
    - Beam quality describes the beam's ability to penetrate
    - Different types of radiation have different beam qualities and can produce different amounts of response
    - Quality factors (QF) are assigned to describe the type of radiation

Type of Radiation	Quality Factor
X-rays, gamma rays, beta particles, electrons	1
Protons	2
Neutrons	3 to 10
Heavy particles (alpha particles)	20

C. Photon, Electron, and Particle Interactions
1. Photon Interactions
    - Photon interactions with electrons can produce coherent or elastic scattering, photoelectric effect, and Compton scattering
        » **Coherent (or elastic) scattering:** the photon interacts with an atomic electron and the photon becomes redirected, or scattered, from its original path without a change in energy
            - Interaction with outer shell electron
            - Low energies and materials with high Z# (atomic number)
            - Usually occurs with energies less than 10 KeV

- » **Photoelectric effect:** the photon is absorbed by an atomic electron and its energy is transferred
  - Results in a photoelectron being ejected from the atom
  - Interaction with inner shell electron
  - Occurs more with-low energy photons interacting with materials with a high Z# (atomic number)
  - Occurs in diagnostic more than therapy
  - Characteristic x-rays are emitted as a result because an outer shell electron has to fill vacancy of the inner shell
- » **Compton scattering:** the photon interacts with an outer shell atomic electron and gives up partial energy before it changes direction
  - Most common interaction in soft tissue in therapy
  - Occurs in energies from 25 keV to 10 MeV
- Photon interactions with atomic nuclei can cause pair production and photonuclear reactions
  - » **Pair production:** incoming photon disappears and then reappears as an electron positron pair
  - » The electron pair becomes two 0.511 MeV photons
    - Threshold energy needed >1.022 MeV
  - » **Photonuclear reactions:** photon goes in and neutron comes out
    - Can occur in high Z# (atomic number) materials such as the jaws or collimators in the head of the linear accelerator
    - Can occur from 7 to 15 MeV
    - Produces neutron radiation in the treatment room with energies greater than 10 MV

2. Electron Interactions
- Electrons are charged particles
- Electrons are directly ionizing and deposit energy in materials they interact with
- Common electron energies are 5 to 20 MeV
- Electrons have two kinds of collisions: elastic and inelastic
- **Elastic collisions:** the total kinetic energy before the collision is the same as the total kinetic energy after the collision
  - » No energy is lost during collisions
- **Inelastic collisions:** some kinetic energy is lost and reappears in another form of energy, like excitation, ionization, bremsstrahlung, etc.
- Electrons travel in a "zigzag" or "tortured" path
- Electrons are easily scattered by high Z# material because of their low mass
- Electron interactions are bremsstrahlung and characteristic
  - » **Bremsstrahlung:** interaction occurs near nucleus
    - Particle slows down as it approaches the nucleus and then changes its direction
  - » **Characteristic:** incoming electron interacts with an inner shell electron, causing the inner shell electron to be ejected
    - An outer shell electron fills the new vacancy

3. Particle Interactions
- Particles are protons, alpha particles, pions, heavy nuclei, etc.
- Heavy charged particles have straight paths
- Particles have a large mass
- Protons are 2,000 times heavier than electrons
- Not easily deflected

D. Elements of Machines Used in Radiation Therapy
1. Linear Accelerator
- The main parts that make up the linear accelerator are the drive stand, gantry, treatment couch, console, electronic cabinet, and modulator cabinet
    - » The modulator cabinet powers the magnetron or klystron
- The three parts of the linear accelerator that can move are the gantry, collimator, and couch
    - » All rotate around the isocenter
- The gantry is attached to the **drive stand**
    - » The drive stand contains the klystron, waveguide, circulator, and cooling system
    - » Linear accelerators need microwaves to help accelerate electrons within the waveguide
    - » Sources of microwaves in a linear accelerator come from a klystron or a magnetron
        - Linear accelerators have either a klystron or a magnetron (never both)
    - » **Klystron:** amplifies microwaves
        - Produces microwaves with a higher power than a magnetron
        - Used in linear accelerators that produce energies above 12 MV
        - Need an "RF driver," which is a source of microwaves
    - » **Magnetron:** generates microwaves
        - Used in machines that only require low energies
    - » **Waveguide:** tube where electrons flow to the gantry under a vacuum
    - » **Circulator:** stop microwaves from being reflected and reentering the klystron
        - Located between the klystron and waveguide
    - » **Modulator:** powers the electron gun and magnetron
    - » **Water-cooling system:** prevents the linear accelerator from overheating
- **Gantry:** directs and aims photons to the patient
    - » **Electron gun:** generates electrons and sends them into the accelerator
        - Made of tungsten
    - » **Accelerator guide:** uses microwaves from klystron to accelerate the electrons to the target
        - Contains sulfur hexafluoride (SF_6) to prevent arcing in the waveguide
    - » **Treatment head:** where the beam shape is formed and the beam output is monitored
        - In photon therapy the components used in the treatment head are (in order): x-ray target, primary collimator, beam-flattening filter, ion chambers, secondary collimators, and slots for wedges, blocks, and compensators
        - In electron therapy the components used in the treatment head are similar, but scattering foils are used instead of the target and flattening filter
        - Scattering foils spread out the electron beam

- There is a magnet system in the gantry that is used to bend electrons 90 to 270 degrees to aim them toward the patient
  - 270-degree magnet system creates a more confined beam than the 90-degree magnet system
- **Ion chambers** are small chambers located in the path of the radiation beam and check the beam's dose rate and symmetry
  - » Most ion chambers are sealed and will not be affected by temperature or pressure
  - » If the ion chambers are unsealed, a correction factor is applied to the output
  - » Positioned after scattering foil (for electron therapy) or flattening filter (for photon therapy)
- During treatments, therapists control and monitor the machine from the control console, which is located outside of the treatment room
- Most newer linear accelerators are calibrated to 100 SAD

2. CT Simulator
- CT simulator consists of the CT scanner and virtual simulation workstation
- External parts of the CT gantry are the controls for couch movements, gantry tilt, emergency off buttons, and localizing lasers
- Internal parts of the CT gantry are the detector array and x-ray tube
- Display uses a matrix size of 512 x 512
- CT creates 3-D images compared with 2-D conventional simulator
- Images can be viewed in the axial, coronal, and sagittal planes
- Images are a display of many small pixels with different shades of gray, depending on the attenuation rate, or Hounsfield units (HU)
  - » -1000 HU = air
  - » 0 HU = water
  - » 1000 HU = dense bone
- CT simulators for radiation therapy have a larger bore than conventional CT
  - » 70 cm or greater
  - » The larger bore size allows for positioning and immobilization devices to fit
- The couch in the CT simulator must be identical to the couch used in the treatment room
- Typical CT simulation slice thickness is 2 to 3 mm
- Spacing between slices should be less than 5 mm
- One CT slice delivers about 1 to 6 cGy at the skin's surface
- Examples of artifacts on the images can be beam hardening, partial volume effect, star artifact, ring artifact, motion, and helical artifacts
- The **window width (WW)** is the spectrum of different shades of gray or contrast on a CT image
- The **window level (WL)** is the average of all the shades of gray in the window width (the median)
- Daily warm-up of the CT simulator includes warming up the x-ray tube, checking if the lasers are in tolerance, scanning a water phantom, and checking for image noise and spatial integrity
  - » Lasers must be positioned within ± 2mm

» Image noise depends on company terms

» Spatial integrity allowance is ± 1 mm

» CT number of water is 0 ± 3 HU

» Field uniformity of water: 5 HU

• Monthly tests check the CT number and compare it to the electron density, reconstruction accuracy, image transfer, and left and right registration

» CT number 0 ± 5 HU

• Annual CT simulator tests check spatial resolution, contrast resolution, and reciprocity of HU numbers with electron density

E. Quality Assurance Tests

1. Warm-up QA of Linear Accelerators and CT Simulators

   a. Interlock Components

   • Machines are either turned off or not able to turn on when conditions are unsafe

   • Provides safety for patient, staff, and machine

   • Linear accelerators have a warm-up timer, which prevents the therapist from turning the beam on until a warm-up is complete and the machine is at an appropriate temperature

   • Door interlock: radiation beam is unable to turn on when the door to the treatment room is open

   » If the door opens while the radiation beam is on, the beam will automatically shut off

   » If this occurs, the beam will not turn back on automatically once the door is closed again

   » The therapist would need to manually turn the beam back on when the door is closed

   » Checked daily

   • Monitor chambers: monitors the dose of the radiation beam and turns beam off when the dose exceeds limits

   • Collision avoidance system: stops motion of the gantry when the head of the gantry is too close to the patient

   » Sensed with a laser or optical guard system on newer Varian machines

   » Other machines, like Elekta, use collision rings

   » Electron cones can detect collision with a mechanical touch guard at the bottom of the cone

      • The collision guard on each cone is checked daily

   • Patient devices like blocks, wedges, and compensators are programmed with a code

   » An interlock will show if the device code does not match the code planned for that specific patient

   • The electron beam cannot be turned on if the electron applicator is not in place

   • Limit switches: stops the gantry, collimator, and couch from moving past the predetermined endpoint

   b. Safety Lights

   • A light turns on when the linear accelerator is on or if a radiation source is exposed

   • Located in several areas: outside of the treatment room, over the treatment door, inside the treatment room, and on the console

» Includes rooms with linear accelerators, HDR units, and Gamma Knife
- A common reason for malfunction is because a light bulb burned out
- Checked daily

c. Emergency Off Buttons
- Emergency switches are switches that terminate the radiation beam and shut down the machine
- Located on the walls of the treatment room, on the linear accelerator, and on the control panel outside of the treatment room
- Switches are checked monthly for safety
- If the emergency switch does not work, the next step would be to use the circuit breaker, which is usually located near the control panel

d. Important Machine Factors
- Cooling water is circulated throughout the linear accelerator to cool internal parts such as the accelerator waveguide, source of microwave power, x-ray target, and bending magnets
- The temperature of the waveguide should be constant at 40 ± 5 °C
  » The microwaves can change with temperature of the metal, so it is important to keep the temperature constant
- Compressed air is used to move the target, control the energy switch, and control the locking system on the carrousel
  » A common pressure used is 45 to 50 psi
- Sulfur hexafluoride (SF_6) is a pressurized gas used to prevent arcing within the waveguide
  » 25 to 32 psi is required

e. Hazards
- Electrical and mechanical hazards can occur if the software within the machine fails
- These may cause injury to the patient, further complications, and possibly death
- Electrical hazards can lead to the wrong dose delivered and the wrong beam energy
- Mechanical hazards can lead to the dose being delivered to the incorrect anatomic location and machine collisions

f. QA of Imaging Mechanics
- Quality control procedures on imaging systems are typically performed by the physicist
- Geometric checks (like alignment between lasers, KV, and MV imagers and the accuracy of couch shifts) are performed monthly
  » ±1mm tolerance
- Image quality checks (like uniformity, noise, spatial resolution and detectability) are performed monthly
  » Less than or equal to 2 mm or 5 lp/cm tolerance
- Imaging dose and generator performance are checked annually

2. Dose Output Verification
  a. *Ways to Measure Beam Output*
    • Beam output can be measured by devices that have multiple ion chambers or diodes
    • Beam outputs can be checked with single ion chambers too
    • Checks beam output on the central axis and off axis
    • Also checks beam flatness and symmetry
      » Checks in transverse and radial directions

  b. *Frequency*
    • Linear accelerator output is checked daily for each beam energy
    • Output tolerance is ±3 percent for electron and photon therapy

  c. *Temperature and Pressure Correction Factor*
    • Temperature and pressure can have an effect on the ion chambers if they are not sealed
    • Pressure and output have a direct relationship
      » As pressure is increased the output is increased
      » As pressure is decreased, the output is decreased
    • Temperature and output have an indirect relationship
      » As temperature is increased, the output is decreased
      » As temperature is decreased, the output is increased
    • Must use a correction factor for temperature and pressure when calculating and measuring dose output if the ion chambers are not sealed
      » Correction factor = $[(T + 273)/295) \times (760 / P)]$
        • T = temperature in Celsius
        • P = pressure

3. Light Field and Treatment Field
  a. *Light and Radiation Field Coincidence Tests*
    • The light field represents the radiation field
    • The light field should be identical to the radiation field
    • Tested with a "ready pack" film, which is a film within a paper covering
      » With the "ready pack" film taped onto the treatment table, the field size is opened to a specific size
      » Trace the corners of the light field so that it can be seen on the film
        • Alternatively, holes can be poked into the corners of the film to designate the light field
      » Then irradiate the film and process it
      » The irradiated field is compared with he markings of the light field
    • Mechanical check with a tolerance of 2 mm
    • Checked monthly
    • Checked after a light bulb has been changed or any other repairs have been made to the light field

b. Collimator Settings
- The field size indicated on the console must match what is projected on the patient
- This can be tested by measuring the field on the table with a ruler at isocenter (100 SAD)
- Test for field sizes ranging from 5x5 cm to 35x35 cm
- Field size tolerance is 2 mm
- Monthly mechanical QA check
- If out of tolerance, this must be repaired by a service engineer before delivering any treatments

c. Multileaf Collimator QA
- Multileaf collimator performance is verified with radiographic imaging
- To verify the calibration of leaf positions, use the picket fence test
  - » Radiograph the MLC leaves 8 times
  - » Each image of the MLCs should be open 5 cm and abut the previous field
  - » Shows if the leaves are misaligned
  - » Also tests the homogeneity of the dose on the match lines
    - Optical density change of ± 20 percent signifies misaligned leaves
  - » According to the Task Group 142 Report, this test should be performed weekly on machines that perform IMRT
- According to the Task Group 142 Report, leaf travel speed and leaf position accuracy for IMRT machines should be performed monthly
  - » Leaf position has a 2 mm tolerance
  - » Speed tolerance is a loss of speed more than 0.5 cm/s
- MLC transmission should be less than 2 percent
  - » Checked annually

d. Laser Accuracy
- Alignment lasers are checked daily
- Lasers must point at and intersect at the isocenter
- Side wall lasers must be collinear
- Tolerance ± 2mm
- Side lasers can be checked by bringing the table up so it is 100 cm from the source (or the calibrated isocenter)
  - » Use the ODI (optical distance indicator)
  - » At this point the lasers must skim the table

4. <u>Gantry and Collimator Rotation</u>

   a. Safety Checks

- To properly check that the gantry rotation for a patient's treatment is safe, a test run (dry run) of the gantry movement should be performed prior to treatment to make sure there are no collisions with the patient, table, or any other devices
- The angle of the gantry or collimator that is displayed should match the actual angle of the gantry or collimator
    - » Checked with a spirit level
    - » Checked with angles at 90-degree intervals
    - » Mechanical check that is performed monthly
    - » Tolerance for gantry and collimator angle is 1 degree

   b. Operating the Gantry

- There are limit switches for the gantry to avoid over rotation of the gantry
- The gantry can be controlled within the room with the pendant or outside of the room at the treatment console when the treatment door is closed

5. <u>Evaluating Quality Assurance Tests</u>

   a. Evaluation

- Mechanical tolerances for linear measurements are typically ± 2 mm
- Tolerances for angles are typically 1 degree
- Dosimetric monthly checks for output have tolerances of 2 percent
- Safety checks are "functional" and either work or don't

   b. What To Do

- When tests fail or are out of tolerance, they must first be repeated
- If they still fail, alert the manager, physicist, and/or service engineer for the machine
- Treatment cannot occur until the issues are fixed
- Record information in accordance with the facility's policies

Part 2: Radiation Protection

A. Radiation Biology

1. Radiosensitivity
   - DNA is the most sensitive part of the cell
     » Located within the nucleus
   - **Law of Bergonie and Tribondeau:** the effects of radiation are greater for cells that divide rapidly, cells that are immature with a long mitotic future, and undifferentiated (have limited purpose other than to divide and replace other cells)
   - **Ancel and Vitemberger:** the extent of radiation damage can change depending on the cell's external factors before, during, or after the delivery radiation
   - The presence of oxygen during a radiation treatment will greatly increase the radiosensitivity of a cell
     » Oxygen enhancement ratio (OER) is 2.5 to 3.0 in human cells
   - On the linear accelerator, lower dose rates cause less damage than higher dose rates
   - High dose rates cause more side effects more rapidly
     » TBI uses high dose rates
   - Therapeutic ratio = (normal tissue tolerance dose) / (tumor lethal dose)
     » Ideally, tumor lethal dose should be less than the normal tissue tolerance dose to avoid damage to healthy tissue

2. Dose-Response Relationships
   - Dose-response relationships are represented by a graph
   - The graph shows information on the cell's response to radiation and cell survival in the presence of radiation
   - There are specific points on the graph that represent important information (D_o, D_q, n)
   - **D_o** (or D_{37}) represents a dose after which only 37 percent of the cell population will survive
     » Cells that are radiosensitive have a low D_o because it takes a lower dose to kill all but 37 percent of the cell population
     » Cells that are radioresistant have a high D_o because it takes a higher dose to kill all but 37 percent of the cell population
   - **Extrapolation number (n)** is the amount of cells or the target number
     » Usually about 2 to 10
   - **D_q** is the quasi-threshold dose, which represents the cells' capability to repair
     » Also known as the shoulder region
     » Graphs with multiple shoulders represent multiple fractions
   - **LET (linear energy transfer)** is the rate that energy is deposited through matter as it travels through it
     » X-rays and gamma rays have a low LET
     » Protons and alpha particles have a high LET
       - On the dose-response relationship graphs, high LET is represented by a steeper curve and a shoulder is either smaller than normal or nonexistent because more cells are killed faster and do not have a chance to repair

47

3. Somatic Effects

- **Stochastic effects** are effects that have a *probability* of occurring depending on the radiation dose
    - » No threshold
    - » Example: cancer
    - » The severity of the effect is specifically related to dose
- **Non-stochastic (deterministic) effects** are effects that occur depending on the *severity* of the radiation dose
    - » There is a threshold
    - » Example: cataracts and erythema
    - » Different doses can cause different effects

a. Effects on Cells

- A **direct effect** is when radiation hits the target (DNA)
- An **indirect effect** is when radiation first hits water within the cell
    - » This leads to radiolysis and free radicals within the cell
    - » A common free radical is hydrogen peroxide (H_2O_2)
    - » Free radicals can then lead to damage of DNA
- Chromosome damage can be single-strand or double-strand breaks
    - » Single-strand breaks can lead to dicentric fragments, acentric fragments, translocation, and/or ring formation
    - » Double-strand breaks can lead to deletions and inversions
- A cell response to radiation is cell death, which is known as apoptosis
- Other cell responses to radiation are division delay, interphase death, and reproductive failure
- The most sensitive cell cycle is the M phase (and also the end of G2)
- Most radioresistant cell cycle is the S phase

b. Effects on Tissues

- The level of response shown by an organ that received radiation depends on the radiation dose, the volume of tissue in the radiation field, the radiosensitivity of the cells involved, and the time that has elapsed since the radiation was delivered
- After radiation damage, organs can **regenerate**, or replace the damaged cells with the same cell type
    - » This can lead to a partial or complete reversal of radiation damage
- After radiation damage, organs can **repair**, or replace the damaged cells with a different cell type
    - » This occurs when parenchymal cells are destroyed
    - » Occurs at doses greater than 1,000 cGy
    - » Can lead to scar formation or fibrosis
- When damage is so great that regeneration and repair are unattainable, necrosis can occur

- Radiation damage is shown quicker in cells with shorter mitotic cycles
  - » Example: skin
  - » Skin reacts more quickly and more severely to radiation compared with more radioresistant organs, such as the lungs
    - By the time the lungs exhibit a reaction, the skin reaction has already healed

c. Effects on the Embryo and Fetus

- The embryo and the fetus are the most radiosensitive stages of human life
- Radiation to the embryo and fetus can be lethal or lead to congenital abnormalities/effects
- If the fetus is exposed to radiation, the effects caused by the radiation are typically present at birth
- If the sperm or ovum is irradiated, the radiation effects may be shown later in life
- When exposure to radiation occurs in the preimplantation stage (day 0 to 10 of gestation), the most common effect is prenatal death
- When exposure occurs during the stage of major organogenesis (day 10 to week 6 of gestation), the most common effects are abnormalities or neonatal death
  - » Some examples of abnormalities are microcephaly, mental retardation, and damage to the skeleton or sensory organs
- The risks of radiation effects are decreased when the fetus is exposed to radiation (week 6 of gestation to birth)

d. Carcinogenesis

- Carcinogenesis is also known as the formation of cancer cells
- This is a stochastic effect and has no threshold
- Any dose of radiation may cause carcinogenesis
- A common example of something that leads to carcinogenesis is radiation

e. Time Dependent Effects

- **Early effects** occur within six months of radiation treatment
  - » Examples: nausea, hair loss, fatigue, and skin erythema
- **Late effects** occur six months after the radiation treatments
  - » Late effects are early changes that have progressed and become irreversible
  - » There is a latent period, or a time between when radiation damage occurs and when radiation effects are shown
  - » Late effects depend on dose per fraction
    - The higher the dose per fraction, the more severe the late effect can be
  - » Examples: fibrosis/scarring, genetic effects, carcinogenicity, leukemia, short life span, cataracts, and telangiectasis (unusual distention of superficial capillaries and arteries)
- **Acute changes** occur when there is damage to and a reduction in the parenchymal cells of the organ
  - » Inflammation, edema, hemorrhage

- Three acute radiation syndromes (total body exposure):
    » **Hematopoietic syndrome** occurs from 100 to 1,000 cGy
        - Mean survival time is 10 to 60 days
        - Most sensitive
    » **Gastrointestinal syndrome** occurs from 1,000 to 10,000 cGy
        - Mean survival time is 4 to 10 days
    » **Cerebrovascular/CNS syndrome** after 10,000 cGy
        - Mean survival time is 0 to 3 days

- **Chronic changes** occur when there is a reduction in non-parenchymal cells, or stromal and vascular cells
    » Fibrosis, atrophy, and ulceration
    » Chronic changes are permanent and cannot be reversed
    » Most severe response of all is necrosis or death
        - $LD_{50/30}$ (50 percent of population dead in 30 days) = 3 to 4 Gy

B. Tissue Tolerances to Radiation

1. Tolerance Doses

- TD 5/5 = the dose of radiation to healthy tissue that will cause a 5 percent chance of complication within five years of the delivered dose
- The following graph shows examples of tolerance doses in cGy and effects by Emami et. Al

Organ	1/3	2/3	3/3	Effect
Esophagus	6,000 cGy	5,800 cGy	5,500 cGy	Stricture/ perforation
Stomach	6,000 cGy	5,500 cGy	5,000 cGy	Ulceration/ perforation
Small Intestine	5,000 cGy	---	4,000 cGy	Obstruction/ perforation/fistula
Colon	5,500 cGy	---	4,500 cGy	Obstruction/ perforation/ ulceration/ fistula
Rectum	---	---	6,000 cGy	Proctitis/necrosis/ fistula
Bladder	---	8,000 cGy	6,500 cGy	Bladder contracture/ volume loss
Femoral Head	---	---	5,200 cGy	Necrosis
TMJ/Mandible	6,500 cGy	6,000 cGy	6,000 cGy	Limited function
Rib Cage	5,000 cGy	---	---	Fracture
Spinal Cord	5 cm/ 5,000 cGy	10 cm/ 5,000 cGy	20 cm/ 4,700 cGy	Myelitis necrosis
Cauda Equine	---	---	6,000 cGy	Nerve damage
Brachial Plexus	6,200 cGy	6,100 cGy	6,000 cGy	Nerve damage
Brain	6,000 cGy	5,000 cGy	4,500 cGy	Nerve damage
Brain Stem	6,000 cGy	5,300 cGy	5,000 cGy	Necrosis/infarction
Optic Nerve	---	---	5,000 cGy	Necrosis/ infarction/ Blindness
Optic Chiasma	---	---	5,000 cGy	Blindness
Eye Lens	---	---	1,000 cGy	Blindness
Eye Retina	---	---	4,500 cGy	Cataracts
Larynx	7,900 cGy	7,000 cGy	7,000 cGy	Cartilage necrosis
Larynx	---	4,500 cGy	4,500 cGy	Laryngeal edema
Parotid	---	3,200 cGy	3,200 cGy	Xerostomia
Lung	4,500 cGy	3,000 cGy	1,750 cGy	Pneumonitis
Heart	6,000 cGy	4,500 cGy	4,000 cGy	Pericarditis
Kidney	5,000 cGy	3,000 cGy	2,300 cGy	Nephritis
Liver	5,000 cGy	3,500 cGy	3,000 cGy	Liver failure
Skin	10 cm2 7,000 cGy	30 cm2 6,000 cGy	100 cm2 5,500 cGy	Telangiectasia/ necrosis/ ulceration
Ear mid/external	3,000 cGy	3,000 cGy	3,000 cGy	Acute serous otitis

2. Fractionation

- **Fractionation** breaks down one large dose into many smaller doses, which encourages the preservation of normal, healthy tissue
  - » Tissues have time to repair themselves between fractions
  - » Not as biologically effective as one large does when irradiating tumors
- The biologic effect of fractionation depends on the four R's
  - » **Repopulation:** remaining cells undergo mitosis and repopulate tissues
    - Unfavorable for malignant tumor cells
    - Favorable in healthy cells within the treatment field
  - » **Redistribution:** remaining cells transition to a different cycle of mitosis after irradiation
  - » **Repair of sublethal damage:** healthy tissues repair the radiation damage when adequate oxygen is available
    - Malignant tumor cells are more hypoxic than normal tissues and therefore they do not easily repair themselves
  - » **Reoxygenation:** hypoxic tumor cells become more oxygenated and therefore more radiosensitive, which allows for more of the tumor to be destroyed
- **OER (oxygen enhancement ratio):** the presence of oxygen makes cells 2.5 to 3 times more sensitive

3. Medical Devices

- Pacemakers are sensitive to radiation and are likely to fail with low doses of radiation
- Pacemakers should never be directly in the path of the radiation beam
  - » Sensitive to scatter as well and should be shielded as best as possible
  - » Typically, manufacturers suggest to keep radiation doses below 500 cGy
- Hearing aids are sensitive to radiation and should be removed before treatment

4. Radiosensitizers and Radioprotectors

- **Radiosensitizers:** substances that increase the response to radiation
  - » Allows for more cells to be killed
  - » Oxygen increases sensitivity the most
  - » Another example is chemotherapy like doxorubicin
- **Radioprotectors:** substances that decrease the response to radiation
  - » Need to be given at the same time as the radiation exposure
  - » Searches for free radicals
  - » Example: sulfhydryls and amifostine
    - Amifostine may also be referred to as Ethyol

C. Radiation Measurements

1. <u>Measurement Systems</u>

    a. *Absorbed Dose (gray)*
    - Unit to describe the amount of energy that has been absorbed in a certain amount of matter
    - The SI unit for the absorbed dose is the Gray (Gy)
    - The traditional unit is the rad
    - 1 Gy = 100 cGy = 100 rad (radiation absorbed dose)
    - 1 rad = 0.01 joule/kg = 100 erg/g
    - 1 Sv = 100 rads = 1 Gy
    - 1 rem = 1 rad

    b. *Dose Equivalent (rem)*
    - A unit that expresses the amount of radiation that is absorbed by a person, while factoring in the biologic effects of the different types of radiation
    - The SI unit for the dose equivalent is the sievert (Sv)
        » Sievert (Sv) = absorbed dose (Gy) x quality factor (QF)
    - Traditional unit is the REM (Roentgen equivalent man)
    - 1 Sv = 100 rem

    c. *Exposure (Roentgen)*
    - Measures the total number of ionizations produced by photons and occur in a unit mass of air (C/kg)
    - 1 R = 2.58 x 10^{-4} Coulomb (C) of charge per kilogram of air
    - Roentgen is only defined at energies lower than 3 MeV

2. <u>Measurement Devices</u>
    - Instruments are used to detect radiation
    - Instruments are calibrated every two years or after any repairs are made

    a. *Ionization Chamber*
    - A gas-filled chamber that has two electrodes with an applied voltage and a meter that measures the electric signal
    - Measures the production of radiation in therapy equipment
        » Within the linear accelerator, ion chambers are the most common way to measure machine output
    - The mass of the gas in the chamber determines the sensitivity of the ion chamber
    - Readings are in mR/hour
    - This instrument is accurate within ± 2 percent
    - The ion chamber usually isn't used for low levels of radiation or radiation contamination because it is not very sensitive
    - When calibrating the ionization chamber, certain correction factors need to be used if the chambers are not sealed
        » Correction factors are temperature, pressure, and volume
        » These factors can cause ionizations

- Examples of ion chambers are a pocket dosimeter and a cutie pie
  - » A pocket dosimeter is a low-energy dosimeter
  - » A cutie pie is a portable ion chamber
    - Determines exposure rate outside the room of a patient with radioactive implants
    - Can detect higher doses than a Geiger-Müller counter

b. Geiger-Müller Detector
- Instrument used to detect radiation of low levels and radioactive contamination
- Very sensitive
- Can detect radiation 100 mrem/hr and less
- This detector responds differently to different photon energies
- GM counter is used to survey rooms for radiation but doesn't actually measure the amount of radiation
- Commonly used to locate sources that have been misplaced

c. TLD/OSL
- Solid-state detectors
- **TLD = thermoluminescent dosimeter:** when heated, this dosimeter lights up in proportion to the amount of radiation that was absorbed
  - » There is a crystal material embedded in the dosimeter
  - » When the crystals are irradiated, electrons are released from their valence bonds and remain trapped within a gap
  - » To get a reading, the dosimeter is heated to about 100°C to 200°C, which sends the electrons back to their valence bonds while releasing characteristic photons (visible light)
  - » TLDs are made of lithium fluoride (LiF) because this material has an atomic number that is very similar to human tissue
  - » Accurate within ± 5 percent
  - » The information can be stored for weeks
  - » Other materials for TLDs are Mg, Ti, and CaF_2
- **OSL = Optically Stimulated Luminescence:** crystals release electrons from their valence bonds when irradiated just like TLDs
  - » However, electrons are released and visible light photons are emitted when they are excited by light instead of heat
  - » Made of aluminum oxide (AL_2O_3:C)

d. Diodes
- Small solid-state detectors
- Very sensitive to radiation
- Can give a real-time reading
- Diodes are the equipment of choice for patient dosimetry because it can measure the beam delivered for treatment
- Diodes are also used for a daily check for the linear accelerator's beam output
- Diodes are not used to calibrate the beam

e. Neutron Detectors
- Important in proton therapy and photon therapy above 10 MV
  - » Neutron scatter occurs at energies above 10 MV

D. Radiation Principles

1. ALARA
- "As low as reasonably achievable"
- An attempt to keep harmful radiation exposure to as little as possible
- This principle assures that the least harm will be done to patients as well as radiation workers
- Radiation workers are at the same risk of death as other workers in "safer" industries
  - » There is no greater risk

2. Methods of Protection
- Decreasing your time spent exposed to radiation reduces the dose received
- Increasing your distance from the source of radiation reduces the dose received
  - » The inverse square law would explain the change in dose with increasing or decreasing distance
  - » Increasing distance is the most efficient way to increase protection
- Proper shielding from radiation is very important in the protection of the radiation worker and the public

E. Monitoring Employees and the General Population

1. NRC Recommendations for personnel monitoring (Report #116) & (Commentary No. 26)

A. Occupational Exposures

1. Effective dose limits

a) Annual	50 mSv (5 rem)
b) Cumulative	10 mSv x age (1 rem x age)

2. Equivalent dose annual limits for tissues and organs

a) Lens of eye	50 mSv (5 rem)
b) Skin, hands, and feet	500 mSv (50 rem)

B. Public Exposures (annual)

1. Continuous/frequent exposure	1 mSv (0.1 rem)
2. Infrequent exposure	5 mSv (0.5 rem)

3. Tissues and organs

a) Lens of eye	15 mSv (1.5 rem)
b) Skin, hands, feet	50 mSv (5 rem)

C. Embryo/Fetus Exposure

1. Total dose	5 mSv (0.5 rem)
2. Monthly effective dose	0.5 mSv (0.05 rem)

2. Employee Records of Radiation Dose
- There is a permanent record of radiation received by the radiation worker
- The radiation worker should be monitored if they are expected to receive more than 10 percent of the effective dose equivalent
- Health care institutions must keep these records forever

F. Monitoring Radiation Areas
1. NRC Regulations
a. Controlled and Uncontrolled Areas
- **Restricted/controlled areas** are areas that are strictly supervised by a radiation safety officer
  - » Usually limited to radiation workers who are monitored for the dose they are receiving
  - » These areas have an occupational limit of radiation and cannot receive more than 1 rem per year
  - » <100 mrem/week or 0.1 rem/week or 1 mSv/week
- **Unrestricted/uncontrolled areas** are areas that are not under the strict supervision of a radiation safety officer
  - » These areas are usually occupied by the general public
  - » Uncontrolled areas cannot receive more than 0.5 rem per year
  - » <1 mSv/week or 2 mrem/week or 0.002 rem/week

b. Necessary Signs for Radiation Areas
- The radiation symbol has three blades that are magenta, purple, or black on a yellow background

 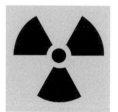

- A **"radiation area"** sign should be posted when a person may receive a dose ≥ 0.005 rem (5 mrem) (0.05 mSv) in one hour at 30 cm from a radiation source
- A sign that reads **"high radiation area"** should be posted when a person can receive a dose ≥ 0.1 rem (1 mSv) in one hour at 30 cm from a radiation source
- A **"very high radiation area"** sign is posted when a person can receive more than 500 rads (5 gray) in one hour at 1 meter from a radiation source
- **"Caution: Radioactive Materials"** is posted in areas where sources of radiation are used and/or stored (example: patient with I-131)

c. Machines Needed for Radiation Detection
- Radiation monitors that are attached to a wall in the entryway of the treatment room
- Signifies when the radioactive source is exposed
- Used for HDR, teletherapy, Co-60 and Gamma Knife Units
- Survey meters may be used as well

2. Radiation Protection for Treatment Rooms
- When designing a radiation therapy treatment room, it should be shielded to protect people from the highest beam energy the machine can produce
- If a machine produces energies above 10 MV, then the room should also be shielded against neutron contamination
- To calculate accurately for shielding, we must take into account the acceptable weekly dose (P), amount of time the beam is on (or the workload, W), portion of time the beam is aimed at a barrier (U), and occupancy (T) of rooms bordering the treatment room
  - $B_p = (Pd^2)/WUT$
  - Use factors are also used to calculate for shielding
    - Floor use factor: 0.31
    - Walls use factor: 0.21
    - Ceiling use factor: 0.26
    - Secondary barrier use factor: 1
- Lead, tungsten, aluminum, and concrete are some materials that are used for barriers
  - Concrete is the most common barrier used and is the cheapest option

a. Primary Barrier
- A wall that is directly hit by the useful/primary radiation beam
- Average thickness of concrete for a primary barrier is 2 meters for beams with energies of 15 to 18 MV

b. Secondary Barrier
- A wall that is hit by scatter or leakage radiation
- Not directly hit by the primary beam
- Average thickness of a secondary concrete barrier is 1 meter for 18 MV energy beams

G. Agencies and Regulations For Handling Radioactive Materials
- **NRC (Nuclear Regulatory Commission)** is a federal agency that regulates the safe use of radioactive materials and protects the public health in regards to radioactive materials
- **EPA (Environmental Protection Agency)** is an agency that regulates the removal, storage, and usage of nuclear waste
- **DOT (Department of Transportation)** helps to supervise and regulate the transportation of hazardous radioactive materials
- Nuclear waste can be disposed of by flushing it into a sewer system after the material has gone through enough decay, by incineration, by burying the material, or by transferring to a person with appropriate authorization
  - To do many of these options, a special license is required
  - Radioactive materials can be disposed of after ten half-lives

Chapter 3: Radiation Therapy Practices

Objectives

- Discuss treatment sites, lymphatic drainage, and metastatic patterns
- Review ways to classify tumors
- Explain the various treatment techniques and immobilization
- Define key concepts in CT simulation
- Identify components of the treatment prescription
- Learn to calculate doses
- Understand the different treatment options
- Review ways to verify the treatment

Part 1: Treatment Sites

A. Information on Different Treatment Sites

1. <u>Brain and Spinal Cord</u>

   - **Anatomy**
     - » The brain has two hemispheres in the cerebrum and two hemispheres in the cerebellum
     - » The brain is protected by cranial bones, meninges, and cerebrospinal fluid
       - • The central nervous system (CNS) has 3 to 5 ounces of cerebrospinal fluid
     - » Ventricles are like chambers or sinuses within the brain that communicate with the canal of the spinal cord and subarachnoid space
       - • Four ventricles: two lateral ventricles, third ventricle, and fourth ventricle
       - • Produce cerebrospinal fluid
     - » CNS is made of gray matter and white matter
       - • Gray matter is made up of supportive nerve cells and makes up the outer portion of the cerebrum
       - • White matter is made up of nerve fibers, axons, and dendrites
     - » The circle of Willis is the main source of blood for the brain
       - • Made up of the internal carotid and vertebral arteries
     - » The spinal cord extends from the medulla oblongata to the filum terminale (L1-L2)
     - » Blood-brain barrier (BBB) protects the brain from toxins
       - • Only substances that are lipid soluble can pass the BBB
       - • Lipid soluble substances are alcohol, nicotine, and heroin
       - • Water-soluble substances may pass if they use a carrier molecule
       - • Water soluble substances are glucose, amino acids, and sodium

   - **Histology**
     - » Gliomas (glioblastoma, astrocytoma, glioblastoma multiforme), medulloblastoma, oligodendroglioma, ependymoma, meningioma, lymphoma, schwannoma
     - » Astrocytoma: most common primary brain tumor in children
     - » Medulloblastoma: second most common primary brain tumor in children
     - » Glioblastoma multiforme: most common primary brain tumor in adults
     - » Overall, the most common brain tumors are metastatic tumors

- **Metastatic patterns**
  - » Most common routes of spread for CNS tumors are local invasion and seeding through cerebrospinal fluid (CFS)
  - » Infrequently metastasize beyond the central nervous system
  - » No metastatic spread via the lymphatic system
  - » Most common area for CSF seeding is in the lumbosacral area

- **Clinical presentation**
  - » "Lhermitte's sign" is a sensation of electrical shock down the neck first and then the extremities
  - » Tumors in different locations exhibit different signs and symptoms
  - » The following image shows the different symptoms that present in different locations of the central nervous system

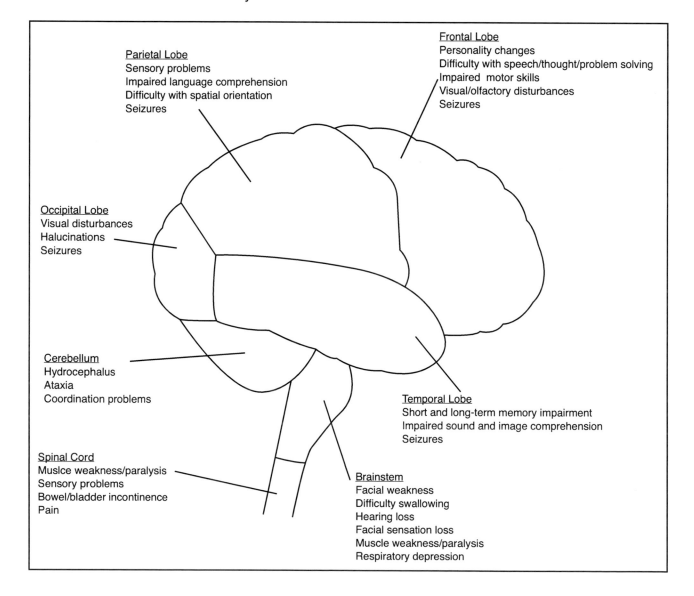

Parietal Lobe
Sensory problems
Impaired language comprehension
Difficulty with spatial orientation
Seizures

Frontal Lobe
Personality changes
Difficulty with speech/thought/problem solving
Impaired motor skills
Visual/olfactory disturbances
Seizures

Occipital Lobe
Visual disturbances
Halucinations
Seizures

Cerebellum
Hydrocephalus
Ataxia
Coordination problems

Spinal Cord
Muslce weakness/paralysis
Sensory problems
Bowel/bladder incontinence
Pain

Temporal Lobe
Short and long-term memory impairment
Impaired sound and image comprehension
Seizures

Brainstem
Facial weakness
Difficulty swallowing
Hearing loss
Facial sensation loss
Muscle weakness/paralysis
Respiratory depression

- **Staging**
  - » GTM (grade, tumor, metastasis)
  - » G1 (well differentiated) to G3 (poorly differentiated)

2. Head and Neck
- **Oral Cavity Anatomy**
  - » Includes lips, buccal mucosa, gingiva, alveolar ridge, hard palate, floor of mouth, retromolar trigone, and anterior two thirds of tongue
  - » Extends from lips to the posterior aspect of the hard palate
  - » Circumvallate papillae separate the anterior two thirds of the tongue, in the oral cavity, from the posterior part of the tongue, which is in the oropharynx
  - » Oral cavity cancers are associated with Plummer-Vinson syndrome (iron deficiency in females)
  - » Cancers of the tongue, floor of mouth, and tonsils are associated with human papillomavirus (HPV)
  - » Lips are the most common site for cancer in the oral cavity
  - » Early signs are poor oral hygiene, poor dental hygiene, nonhealing ulcers, leukoplakia, and erythroplasia
- **Oral Cavity Pathology**
  - » Majority are squamous cell carcinoma (SCC)
  - » Some can be verrucous SCC or spindle cell SCC
- **Oral Cavity Lymphatics**
  - » Upper lip drains into the submandibular and preauricular nodes
  - » Lower lip and anterior mouth drain to submental nodes
  - » Oral tongue drains to the anterior cervical chain nodes
  - » Buccal mucosa drains to the submandibular and subdigastric nodes
- **Oral Cavity Spread Patterns**
  - » Lymphatic and blood-borne spread is rare
  - » Most common site of spread is cervical lymph nodes

- **Pharynx Anatomy**
  - » Three subdivisions in order from superior to inferior: nasopharynx, oropharynx, hypopharynx/laryngopharynx
  - » Cancers in the pharynx have symptoms, such as consistent sore throat, pain while swallowing, pain in the ear, and cervical node enlargement
  - » **Nasopharynx:**
    - Positioned posterior to the nose and extends inferiorly to the uvula
    - Level of C1
    - Tumors in this region are hard to reach in surgery
    - Located close to the base of the brain
    - Carcinomas usually occur in the lateral walls of the nasopharynx
    - There is a connection between nasopharyngeal cancers and the Epstein-Barr virus (EBV)
    - Adenoids are located within the nasopharynx

» **Oropharynx:**
  - Positioned posterior to the oral cavity and extends from the soft palate to the hyoid bone
  - Level of C2 to C3
  - Contains lymphoid tissue called palatine tonsils
  - Most cancers in the oropharynx occur in the tonsils
» **Laryngopharynx:**
  - Extends from the hyoid bone to the esophagus
  - Epiglottis is the superior border at the level of C3
  - Located C3 to C6
  - Posterior to the larynx
  - Made up of the pyriform sinuses, postcricoid and lower posterior pharyngeal walls
  - Piriform sinus is the most common location for cancer within the hypopharynx

- **Pharynx Pathology**
  » Majority are squamous cell carcinoma (SCC)
- **Pharynx Lymphatics**
  » Oropharynx drains to subdigastric, upper cervical, submaxillary and parapharyngeal nodes
  » Nasopharynx drains to cervical nodes, retropharyngeal node (node of Rouvière), and jugulodigastric node
  » Hypopharynx drains to midcervical nodes, superior deep, middle and low jugular nodes; and retropharyngeal node (node of Rouvière)
- **Pharynx Spread Patterns**
  » Oropharynx: spread to lymph nodes (ipsilateral and/or contralateral) and invade structures located close to the tumor
  » Nasopharynx: cranial nerve involvement is common, as is metastasis to bone, lung or liver
  » Hypopharynx: commonly spreads to lymph nodes and invades nerves and muscles nearby

- **Larynx Anatomy**
  » Extends from the epiglottis to the cricoid cartilage (C3 to C6)
  » Includes the glottis, supraglottis, and subglottis
    - Glottis = true vocal cords
  » 5 cm long and made up of six different pieces of cartilage
  » Cancer in the larynx is strongly associated with cigarette smoking
  » HPV is related to laryngeal cancers
  » Common symptoms are constant soreness of the throat and hoarseness
- **Larynx Pathology**
  » Majority are squamous cell carcinomas

- **Larynx Lymphatics**
  - » Glottic cancers rarely spread to lymph nodes and have small treatment fields (5x5 cm or 6x6 cm)
  - » If a glottic cancer were to spread, it would most likely go to the subdigastric node
  - » Supraglottic cancers spread to the spinal accessory chain of lymph nodes
- **Larynx Spread Patterns**
  - » Main spread is to local lymph nodes or to the supraclavicular nodes

- **Salivary Gland Anatomy**
  - » Three main pairs of salivary glands (parotid, submandibular, and sublingual glands)
  - » The parotid is the largest of all salivary glands
    - Located anterior and inferior to ear and is superficial
    - Opens into the oral cavity
    - Most common salivary gland cancer occurs in the parotid glands
    - Can be treated with a wedge-pair technique
  - » Most of these cancers present as a rapidly growing mass
- **Salivary Gland Pathology**
  - » Parotid gland cancers are mostly adenocarcinoma
  - » Other malignant types are adenoid cystic and mucoepidermoid
  - » Most tumors in the major salivary glands are benign
- **Salivary Gland Lymphatics**
  - » Spread to nodes on the same side (ipsilateral) as the tumor
  - » Spread to nodes in the facial group, submandibular group, and extraglandular parotid group
- **Salivary Gland Spread Patterns**
  - » Tumors can involve cranial, facial nerves, and arteries within the neck

- **Thyroid Anatomy**
  - » Right and left lobes connected by an isthmus
  - » Located close to the larynx, trachea, and esophagus
  - » Supports metabolism and creates hormones
  - » Radiation exposure is believed to be a cause of thyroid cancer
  - » Thyroid cancers may present as a palpable mass
- **Thyroid Pathology**
  - » Papillary, follicular, medullary, and anaplastic
  - » Most common are papillary, mixed papillary-follicular, and follicular
    - Can be treated with I-131
- **Thyroid Lymphatics**
  - » Internal jugular chain, anterior cervical node (Delphian node), pretracheal nodes, and paratracheal nodes

- **Thyroid Spread Patterns**
  - » Papillary and mixed papillary-follicular cancers spread through lymph nodes
  - » Follicular cancers spread through the blood stream to bone, lungs, liver and brain
  - » Medullary cancers spread regionally and to cervical lymph nodes
    - Distant metastasis to lungs, liver, and bone
  - » Anaplastic cancers spread locally to skin and trachea and to lymph nodes

- **Head and Neck Lymphatics**
  - » Jugulodigastric lymph node = subdigastric node
    - Located below mastoid tip
    - Receives almost all lymph from the head and neck area
    - Commonly involved in the treatment fields
  - » Node of Rouvière = lateral retropharyngeal node
    - Included in treatment fields
    - Difficult or impossible to reach in surgery, which leads to a high risk of distant metastasis
  - » Spinal accessory chain = posterior cervical lymph node chain
  - » Mastoid node = retroauricular node

3. Breast
- **Anatomy**
  - » The breast is made up of 15 to 20 lobes, adipose tissue, connective tissue, circulatory vessels, lymphatic vessels, and nerves
  - » The lobes produce milk and drain to the nipple
  - » The nipple is encircled by a pigmented area called the areola
  - » The breast is positioned between 2nd and 6th rib and from the sternum to the midaxillary line
  - » The Tail of Spence refers to the breast tissue that is close to the axilla
  - » Muscles that are underneath the breast are the pectoralis major and serratus anterior muscles
    - Other muscles close to the breast are the pectoralis minor and the latissimus dorsi
  - » Cooper's suspensory ligaments are connective tissue that extend throughout the breast to help support it
  - » Most common site for breast cancer is the upper outer quadrant (UOQ)
  - » Chemotherapy used for breast cancer is CMF (cyclophosphamide, methotrexate, and 5-FU)

- **Lymphatics**
  - » Involvement of lymph is important in prognosis
  - » Superficial lymph nodes in the breast are in the skin overlying the breast
  - » Deep lymph in the breast are the axillary, internal mammary (IM) and supraclavicular lymph nodes
  - » Axillary lymph nodes: main site of drainage from the ipsilateral breast
    - 10 to 38 nodes in each axilla

- Three main sections (levels I, II, and III)
- Level I: lowest and most superficial; first place for drainage; located lateral to the pectoralis minor muscle
- Level II: located under the pectoralis minor muscle; more superior than level I
- Level III: more superior than level II; located superior to the pectoralis minor muscle
  » Internal mammary lymph nodes: located lateral to the sternum on each side
- Located in the first through third intercostal spaces
- Average amount of IM nodes is eight
- Four nodes on each side of the sternum
  » Supraclavicular lymph nodes: above clavicle
- Less common site for nodal spread

- **Pathology**
  » Most common is infiltrating ductal carcinoma
  » Infiltrating lobular carcinoma is the second most common histopathology of breast cancer
  » Ductal or lobular carcinoma in situ means that the cancer cells did not invade the basement membrane
  » Inflammatory breast cancer is very rare
- 1 percent of all cases
- Clinical presentation is peau d'orange, erythema, thickening, warmth, and hardening of the breast
- Very poor prognosis with a survival time of less than two years
  » Male breast cancer is less than 1 percent of all breast cancer cases

- **Spread Patterns**
  » Breast cancer spreads slowly
  » Invades locally through direct extension within the same breast
  » Regional involvement spreads to the axillary and IM nodes
- Lymph nodes can demonstrate skip metastasis
- Not in direct order (higher nodes may be positive for disease before some lower nodes are)
- If IM nodes and supraclavicular nodes have disease, the prognosis is worse
  » Common sites of distant metastasis is to sites such as bone, lung, brain, or liver
- T-spine is the common location for bone metastasis
  » Spreads through the Batson venous plexus to the skin

4. Lung
- **Anatomy**
  » Right lung has three lobes and is shorter and wider than the left lung, which has two lobes
  » The lungs are lined by two membranes called the pleura
- Visceral pleura lines the surface of the lung

- Parietal pleura lines the thoracic wall
- Space between the pleura is called the pleural cavity
» The carina is where the trachea bifurcates and is located around T4 to T5
» The trachea divides into the primary bronchi, then to the secondary bronchi, then to the tertiary bronchi, then to the bronchioles, then to alveolar ducts
- Alveolar ducts are where oxygen and carbon dioxide are exchanged
» The hilum is where blood vessels, lymphatic vessels, and nerves gain entry to the lungs
» Main symptom of lung cancer is a cough
» A Pancoast tumor occurs when the tumor is in the apex of the lung and the patient experiences pain in the shoulder and arm, muscle atrophy, and Horner syndrome
» Superior vena cava syndrome occurs when the tumor compresses the superior vena cava, which makes it difficult for the patient to breathe

- **Lymphatics**
  » Main method of regional spread of lung cancer
  » All lymph involved with the lung drains into the intrapulmonary nodes
  » Bronchopulmonary nodes, hilar nodes, interlobar nodes, and mediastinal nodes
  - Superior mediastinal nodes are the paratracheal, pretracheal, the retrotracheal nodes and the azygos nodes
  - Inferior mediastinal nodes are the subcarinal, paraesophageal and pulmonary ligament nodes

- **Pathology**
  » Small cell lung cancer (SCLC) and non-small cell lung cancer (NSCLC)
  » Small cell lung cancer is also called oat cell and includes anaplastic carcinomas
  - High mortality rate and very aggressive
  - Metastasizes early to the brain, therefore prophylactic cranial irradiation is sometimes used
  - Connected with tobacco use
  - Located centrally near the proximal bronchi
  - More common in men
  » Non-small cell lung cancers include adenocarcinoma, large cell carcinoma and epidermoid/squamous cell carcinoma
  - Adenocarcinomas are not connected with tobacco use
  - Located toward the periphery of the lungs
  - More common in women
  - Better prognosis than SCLC
  » Mesothelioma occurs in the lining of the lungs
  - Connected to asbestos exposure
  - Occurs less frequently compared with NSCLC & SCLC

- **Spread patterns**
  - » Tumor can extend locally to other locations in the lung and organs nearby like the ribs, heart, esophagus, and vertebrae
  - » Common route of spread is through lymphatics
  - » Distant spread occurs through the circulatory system
    - • Can spread to distant sites like the liver, brain, bones, bone marrow, adrenal glands, kidneys, cervical lymph nodes, and contralateral lung

5. Abdomen, Pelvis, Gastrointestinal, and Genitourinary, etc.
- **Esophagus Anatomy**
  - » Muscular tube located between the pharynx and the stomach
  - » Starts after the cricoid cartilage around C6 and ends at around T10
  - » 25 cm in length
  - » Three divisions: upper third, middle third, lower third
  - » Posterior to the trachea
  - » Made up of three layers: mucosa, submucosa, and muscular layer
  - » Common symptoms are dysphagia (difficulty swallowing) and weight loss
- **Esophagus Lymphatics**
  - » There are lymphatic vessels within the walls of the esophagus
  - » Lymphatic spread can demonstrate skip metastasis
  - » Upper third of the esophagus drains to the internal jugular, cervical, paraesophageal, and supraclavicular nodes
  - » Middle third of the esophagus drains to the paratracheal, hilar, subcarinal, paraesophageal, and paracardial nodes
  - » Lower third of the esophagus drains to the celiac axis, gastric nodes, and nodes within the lesser curvature of the stomach
- **Esophagus Pathology**
  - » Squamous cell carcinomas are common in the upper and middle sections of the esophagus
  - » Adenocarcinomas are common in the lower section of the esophagus and GE junction
    - • Adenocarcinoma is the most common esophageal cancer
- **Esophagus Spread Patterns**
  - » Skip lesions are possible
  - » Can invade organs that are close by
  - » Distant spread is common to the liver and lungs

- **Stomach Anatomy**
  - » Located in the upper left region of the abdomen
  - » Four regions: cardiac, fundic, body, and pyloric
  - » Has a lesser curvature on the medial side and a greater curvature on the lateral side

- **Stomach Lymphatics**
  - » Celiac nodes, splenic hilum, suprapancreatic nodal group, porta hepatis, and nodes in the gastroduodenal area
- **Stomach Pathology**
  - » Majority are adenocarcinoma
  - » Can also be a lymphoma (poor prognosis)
- **Stomach Spread Patterns**
  - » Can spread through direct extension to nearby organs such as the omenta, pancreas, diaphragm, transverse colon, and duodenum
  - » Distant spread is common to the liver and lungs

- **Small Bowel Anatomy**
  - » Starts at the pyloric sphincter and ends at the ileocecal valve
  - » The walls consist of four layers: mucosa, submucosa, muscle layer, and serosa
  - » Villi are extensions of the mucosa that absorb nutrients
  - » Three sections listed in order: duodenum, jejunum, and ileum
- **Small Bowel Lymphatics**
  - » Mesenteric and celiac nodes
- **Small Bowel Pathology**
  - » Adenocarcinoma
- **Small Bowel Spread Patterns**
  - » Liver is the most common site of distant spread

- **Large Bowel Anatomy**
  - » Starts at the ileocecal valve and ends at the anus
  - » Colon divided into eight regions (listed in order): cecum, ascending colon, hepatic flexure, transverse colon, splenic flexure, descending colon, sigmoid, and rectum
  - » Parts of the large intestine that are intraperitoneal are the cecum, transverse colon, and sigmoid
  - » Parts of the large intestine that are retroperitoneal are the ascending and descending colon and the hepatic and splenic flexures
  - » The walls consist of four layers: mucosa, submucosa, muscle layer, serosa
  - » Types of surgery on the colorectal area are anterior resection and abdominoperineal resection
    - **Anterior resection:** removes colon, but leaves the sphincter and rectum
    - **Abdominoperineal resection (APR):** removes the anus and part of rectum
  - » Familial adenomatous polyposis (FAP): genetic disorder of the colorectal area
    - Multiple benign polyps may develop as a teen and have a possibility in becoming malignant if they are not removed
  - » Uses Dukes staging system and modified Astler-Coller (MAC) classification

- **Large Bowel Lymphatics**
  - » Right colon drains to the ileocecal and right colic nodes
  - » Left colon drains to the mid-colic, inferior mesenteric, and left colic nodes
  - » Sigmoid colon drains to the inferior mesenteric nodes and nodes that run alongside the superior rectal, sigmoidal, and sigmoidal mesenteric vessels
  - » Upper rectum drains to nodes that follow along the middle rectal vessels
  - » Middle and lower rectum drain to internal iliac nodes
  - » Lower rectal and anal canal drain into the inguinal nodes
  - » Other nodes involved in rectal cancer are the perirectal, lateral sacral, and presacral nodes

- **Large Bowel Pathology**
  - » Adenocarcinoma is the most common
  - » Mucinous adenocarcinoma, signet-ring cell carcinoma, and squamous cell carcinoma
- **Large Bowel Spread Patterns**
  - » Spread locally via direct extension in a radial style
  - » Liver is the most common site of distant spread
  - » Can also spread distally to the lung
  - » Peritoneal seeding may also occur

- **Anus Anatomy**
  - » Anal canal is about 3 to 4 centimeters
  - » Starts at the anal verge, where the rectum meets the anus
  - » Most common symptom of anal cancer is rectal bleeding
- **Anus Lymphatics**
  - » Cancers spread to the lymph nodes early on
  - » First locations of lymphatic spread are the perirectal and anorectal nodes
  - » Cancers that spread above the dentate line can spread to the internal iliac nodes and lateral sacral nodes
  - » Cancers below the dentate line may spread to the inguinal lymph nodes
- **Anus Pathology**
  - » Most common is squamous cell carcinoma
  - » Other types are basiloid or cloacogenic cancer, adenocarcinomas, mucoepidermoid, melanomas, and basal cell carcinomas
- **Anus Spread Patterns**
  - » Most common is direct extension
  - » Distant metastasis occurs in the liver or lungs

- **Pancreas Anatomy**
  - » Located behind the peritoneum in the upper abdomen
  - » Located around L1 to L2
  - » The head of the pancreas is located to the right, within the loop of the duodenum
    - • The head of the pancreas is the most common site for cancer
  - » The tail of the pancreas is located to the left and next to the spleen
  - » The islets of Langerhans secrete hormones such as insulin and glucagon
  - » Common surgery for pancreatic cancer is the Whipple procedure (pancreaticoduodenectomy), which removes part of the pancreas, small intestine, and gallbladder
- **Pancreas Lympatics**
  - » Superior pancreaticoduodenal node, inferior pancreaticoduodenal node, porta hepatis node, celiac nodes, and superior mesenteric nodes
- **Pancreas Pathology**
  - » Majority are adenocarcinomas
  - » Other types of pancreatic cancers are islet cell tumors, acinar cell carcinomas, and cystadenocarcinomas
- **Pancreas Spread Patterns**
  - » Pancreatic cancers invade locally to lymph or to organs nearby such as the duodenum, stomach, or colon
  - » A common location of distant spread is to the liver or peritoneal seeding

- **Adrenal Anatomy**
  - » Paired glands that are located above the kidneys
  - » The cortex is the outer part that produces steroid hormones
  - » The medulla is the inner part that produces epinephrine
- **Adrenal Lymphatics**
  - » Paraaortic nodes
- **Adrenal Pathology**
  - » Adrenocortical tumors and adrenal medulla-pheochromocytomas
- **Adrenal Spread Patterns**
  - » Invade locally to nearby organs
  - » Distant spread to paraaortic nodes, lungs, liver, or brain
  - » Tumors of the right adrenal gland commonly spread to the kidney, liver, or vena cava
  - » Tumors of the left adrenal gland commonly spread to the kidney, pancreas, or diaphragm

- **Liver Anatomy**
  - » Largest gland in the body
  - » Two lobes on the anterior surface (right lobe and left lobe)
  - » Two lobes on the visceral surface (caudate lobe and quadrate lobe)
  - » Kupffer cells in the liver are responsible for cleaning the blood
  - » The liver produces bile

- **Liver Lymphatics**
  - » Celiac nodes, porta hepatic nodes, cystic nodes, and hilar nodes
- **Liver Pathology**
  - » Most common type is hepatocellular carcinoma
- **Liver Spread Patterns**
  - » Invades locally within the liver or to the portal and hepatic veins
  - » Spreads distantly to the lung or brain

- **Gallbladder Anatomy**
  - » Pear-shaped pouch that is located on the visceral surface of the liver
  - » Stores bile and empties it into the duodenum when stimulated
- **Gallbladder Lymphatics**
  - » Celiac nodes
  - » Lymph nodes within the porta hepatis and pancreaticoduodenal groups
- **Gallbladder Pathology**
  - » Most common type is adenocarcinoma
- **Gallbladder Spread Patterns**
  - » Common areas of spread are the liver, peritoneal seeding, and lungs
  - » Less common spread is to the ovaries, spleen, or bones

- **Ureter Anatomy**
  - » Small tubes that descend from the kidneys to the urinary bladder
  - » Parallel to the psoas muscles
  - » 25 cm long and located in the retroperitoneal space
  - » Brings urine from the renal pelvis to the bladder
- **Ureter Lymphatics**
  - » Renal hilar, paraaortic, paracaval, common iliac, internal iliac, and external iliac nodes
- **Ureter Pathology**
  - » Transitional cell carcinomas
  - » Squamous cell carcinomas are possible, but more rare
- **Ureter Spread Patterns**
  - » Direct extension or hematogenous spread

- **Kidney Anatomy**
  - » Located from around T12 to L3 in the retroperitoneal space
  - » Two kidneys, each located on either side of the spine
  - » Right kidney is lower than the left kidney
  - » Filters blood
- **Kidney Lymphatics**
  - » Right kidney drains to paracaval and interaortocaval lymph nodes
  - » Left kidney drains to the paraaortic lymph nodes

- **Kidney Pathology**
  - » Renal cell carcinomas, adenocarcinoma, clear cell carcinoma, and granular cell carcinoma
- **Kidney Spread Patterns**
  - » Direct extension through renal capsule
  - » Distant metastasis to lung, soft tissue, bone, liver, skin, or central nervous system

- **Bladder Anatomy**
  - » Located in true pelvis when completely emptied
  - » The apex of the bladder is located inferiorly and points to the pubic symphysis
  - » The trigone is on the posterior wall of the bladder and formed from three openings from the two ureters and the urethra
  - » Cancers are commonly found in the trigone, lateral walls, posterior walls, and the neck of the bladder
- **Bladder Lymphatics**
  - » External iliac, common iliac, presacral and paraaortic nodes
- **Bladder Pathology**
  - » Transitional cell carcinoma is the most common
  - » Others: squamous cell carcinoma, adenocarcinoma, and small cell carcinoma
- **Bladder Spread Patterns**
  - » Distant metastasis to the lung, bone, or liver

- **Urethra Anatomy**
  - » Female urethra is 4 cm in length
  - » Male urethra is longer and extends from the bladder to the external urethral meatus
- **Urethra Lymphatics**
  - » Entire urethra drains to the obturator, internal iliac, and external iliac nodes
  - » Urethral meatus drains to the superficial inguinal, deep inguinal, and external iliac nodes
- **Urethra Pathology**
  - » Squamous cell cancers
- **Urethra Spread Patterns**
  - » Direct extension

6. Reproductive Systems
  - **Prostate Anatomy**
    - » A gland that surrounds the male urethra
    - » Solid organ that is shaped like a walnut
    - » Located after the bladder and before the urogenital diaphragm
    - » The prostate is attached to and posterior to the pubic symphysis
    - » Prostate screening test is the PSA (prostate specific antigen)
      - Normal range is less than or equal to 4 ng/mL

- » Prostate cancers use Gleason grading
  - • Graded 1 to 5 (well differentiated to poorly differentiated)
  - • Takes scores from two different locations in the prostate and adds them together
- **Prostate Lymphatics**
  - » Periprostatic, obturator, external iliac, hypogastric, common iliac, and periaortic nodes (in order of spread)
  - » Paraaortic nodes are involved with metastasis
- **Prostate Pathology**
  - » Most common is adenocarcinoma
- **Prostate Spread Patterns**
  - » Distant spread is rare but can go to the bones, liver, or lungs
  - » The spine is the most common location of bone metastasis
  - » Can spread through direct extension to seminal vesicles, bladder, or rectum

- **Testes Anatomy**
  - » The testes are located within the scrotum and attached by the spermatic cords
  - » Left testis is longer than the right testis
  - » Testes hold the spermatozoa and produce testosterone
  - » Cryptorchidism leads to an increased risk for testicular cancer
  - » A common symptom is a painless swelling or mass
- **Testes Lymphatics**
  - » Left side drains to the left renal hilum nodes
  - » Right side drains to the pericaval nodes
    - • Cancers on the right side may cross over to the left renal hilum nodes after spreading to the primary nodes
  - » Skin of testes drain to the inguinal nodes
- **Testes Pathology**
  - » Majority are germ cell tumors
  - » Seminomas or nonseminomatous germ cell tumors
    - • Types of seminomas: classic, anaplastic, and spermatocytic
    - • Types of nonseminomatous tumors: embryonal carcinoma teratoma, choriocarcinoma, and yolk sac tumor
- **Testes Spread Patterns**
  - » Seminomas usually remain local and only involve lymph nodes
  - » Seminomas spread in an order
  - » Hematogenous spread of seminomas is rare but can spread to lung, bone, liver, and brain
  - » Nonseminomatous tumors are more radioresistant and more likely to involve nodes and metastasize through hematogenous spread
  - » Nonseminomatous tumors can have distant spread to lungs or liver

- **Endometrium Anatomy**
  - » Endometrium lines the uterus
  - » Innermost layer of the uterus
    - The uterus is a muscular organ located in the pelvis, between the rectum and the bladder
  - » Made up of columnar cells
  - » Taking the drug tamoxifen increases the risk of endometrial cancer
  - » A common clinical presentation is postmenopausal vaginal bleeding
  - » Endometrial cancer is the most common gynecologic malignancy
  - » Uses FIGO staging system
- **Endometrium Lymphatics**
  - » Internal and external iliac pelvic nodes; paraaortic nodes
- **Endometrium Pathology**
  - » Most common is adenocarcinoma
  - » Others: adenocarcinoma with squamous differentiation, papillary serous adenocarcinoma, clear cell adenocarcinoma, and sarcomas
- **Endometrium Spread Patterns**
  - » Spreads to the myometrium
  - » Direct extension to the cervix, vagina, parametrial tissue, bladder, or rectum
  - » Peritoneal seeding and hematogenous spread can happen, but are rare

- **Cervix Anatomy**
  - » Narrow section inferior to the uterus and superior to the vagina
  - » The internal os is the opening between the body of the uterus and the cervix
  - » The external os is the opening from the cervix leading into the vagina
  - » Uses FIGO staging system
  - » Cancer detected by the Papanicolaou (Pap) smear
  - » Common clinical presentations are post-coital bleeding, increased menstrual bleeding, and painful intercourse
  - » Important points for high dose rate (HDR) treatments:
    - *POINT A*: 2 cm superior to the cervical os and 2 cm lateral to the endocervical canal
    - *POINT B*: 3 cm lateral to point A
- **Cervix Lymphatics**
  - » Internal iliac, external iliac, and obturator nodes
  - » Distant spread to paraaortic, mediastinal, and supraclavicular nodes
- **Cervix Pathology**
  - » Squamous cell carcinoma
  - » Others: adenocarcinoma, clear cell carcinoma
- **Cervix Spread Patterns**
  - » Metastatic spread to the lungs, bones, or liver
  - » Direct extension to the bladder or rectum

- **Ovaries Anatomy**
  - » Paired and located on either side of the uterus
  - » Most deadly gynecologic cancer
  - » Patients usually have very few symptoms until later stages
  - » Common symptoms are abdominal pain, pelvic pain, abdominal distention, and gastrointestinal symptoms
  - » Serum CA-125 is elevated when ovarian carcinoma is present
  - » Common in older women ages 50 to 70
  - » The use of oral contraceptives and having children help to decrease the risk of ovarian cancer
  - » Uses FIGO staging system
- **Ovaries Lymphatics**
  - » Primarily spread to the periaortic nodes
  - » Can also spread to the external iliac and inguinal nodes
- **Ovaries Pathology**
  - » Most common is epithelial
  - » Others: serous cystadenocarcinoma, germ cell, sex cord, or stromal tumors
- **Ovaries Spread Patterns**
  - » Abdominal seeding
  - » Distant spread to lungs

- **Vagina Anatomy**
  - » Muscular tube about 7.5 inches long
  - » Posterior to the bladder and anterior to the rectum
  - » Most common location of vaginal cancers is on the posterior wall of the upper third of the vagina
  - » Clinical presentation is vaginal bleeding
  - » Uses FIGO staging system
- **Vagina Lymphatics**
  - » Most common node involved is the inguinal node
- **Vagina Pathology**
  - » Most common are squamous cell carcinomas
  - » Malignant melanomas, sarcomas, malignant lymphomas, and clear cell adenocarcinomas
    - Clear cell carcinoma occurs in some women who were exposed to the drug diethylstilbestrol (DES) in utero
- **Vagina Spread Patterns**
  - » Direct extension to nearby tissues
  - » Squamous cell carcinomas spread to the lungs, liver, or supraclavicular nodes

- **Vulva Anatomy**
  - » Mons pubis, clitoris, labia majora, labia minora, and vaginal vestibule
  - » Most cancers occur in the labia majora and minora
  - » Common clinical presentation is a mass
  - » Uses FIGO staging system
- **Vulva Lymphatics**
  - » Superficial inguinal, superficial and deep femoral, and external and common iliac nodes
  - » Cloquet's node
- **Vulva Pathology**
  - » Squamous cell carcinoma is the most common
  - » Others: adenocarcinomas
- **Vulva Spread Patterns**
  - » Distant spread to lung, liver, or bone

7. Skeletal
- **Anatomy**
  - » Skeletal system is made of bones and cartilage
  - » Most skeletal cancers are metastatic
  - » Most tumors originate in the mesoderm, primitive mesenchyme, and ectoderm cells
  - » Tumors commonly occur in areas where rapid growth is occurring, such as the growth plate
    - • Most tumors occur in the distal femur and proximal tibia because they have the largest growth plates
  - » The diaphysis of a long bone is the main shaft
  - » The epiphyses are two knob-like portions of the bone at either end
  - » The periosteum is the hard covering on the bone
  - » Common sites for osteosarcomas: distal femur, proximal tibia, and proximal humerus
  - » Common sites for chondrosarcomas: femur, shoulder girdle, and proximal humerus
  - » Common sites for malignant fibrous histocytomas (MFH) or fibrosarcomas: long, tubular bones like the femur or tibia
  - » Common sites for Ewing's sarcoma: lower half of the body in the diaphysis of the bone
  - » Common sites for metastatic tumors: vertebral bodies, pelvic bones, and ribs
  - » Pain is the most common clinical presentation of bone tumors

- **Lymphatics**
  - » Lymphatic spread is not common unless the tumor occurs in the trunk of the body
  - » Lower limb and lower half of trunk drain to femoral nodes
  - » Upper limb and upper half of trunk drain to axillary nodes
  - » Skull and facial bones drain to neck nodes

- **Pathology**
  - » Osteosarcomas, chondrosarcomas, fibrosarcomas, MFH, Ewing's sarcoma, etc.
  - » Osteosarcoma is the most common bone tumor

- **Spread Patterns**
  - » Commonly spreads through the blood to the lungs
  - » May spread to the bone, liver, or brain
  - » Skip metastasis is common for osteosarcomas

8. Lymphoma (Hodgkin's and Non-Hodgkin's)
  - The lymphatic system comprises lymphatic vessels, organs, and fluid called lymph
  - Functions of the lymphatic system: drain interstitial fluid and filter foreign substances and cellular waste; absorb fats and transport them to the bloodstream; provide immunity to the body by trying to defend against infectious and foreign organisms
  - Lymphatic vessels eventually empty into the thoracic duct or the right lymphatic duct, which then drains into the subclavian veins
  - Lymphatic organs are the spleen, thymus, tonsils, and thoracic duct
    - » The spleen is the largest of the lymphatic organs
  - Major lymph nodes:
    - » **Waldeyer's ring:** tonsillar lymphatic that surrounds the nasopharynx and oropharynx
    - » Cervical, preauricular, occipital, axillary, hilar, mediastinal, paraaortic, iliac, inguinal, and femoral lymph nodes
  - Peyer's patches are lymphatic tissue in the ileum on the small intestine
  - T cells are in the thymus
  - B cells are in the bone marrow

- **Hodgkin's lymphoma**
  - » The Reed-Sternberg cells are present in lymph nodes
  - » Reed-Sternberg cells determine whether lymphoma is Hodgkin's or non-Hodgkin's lymphoma
    - This cell is a giant connective tissue cell that is binucleate
  - » Associated with the Epstein-Barr virus (EBV)
  - » Hodgkin's lymphoma has a predictable, contiguous spread pattern throughout the lymph
  - » Occurs in bimodal age-groups
    - Approximately 25 to 30 years old and 75 to 80 years old
  - » Common clinical presentation is a painless mass found by the patient
    - Usually in the neck or supraclavicular regions
  - » Some patients also present with B symptoms:
    - Fever, night sweats, and 10 percent weight loss within six months
    - Patients with B symptoms have a worse prognosis
  - » Chemotherapy used to treat Hodgkin's lymphoma: MOPP (nitrogen mustard, vincristine sulfate [Oncovin], procarbazine hydrochloride, and prednisone) and ABVD (adriamycin, bleomycin, vinblastine, and dacarbazine)
  - » Radiation therapy technique used is called the mantle

- » **Pathology**
  - Nodular lymphocyte predominant Hodgkin's lymphoma (NLPHL)
  - Classic Hodgkin's lymphoma (CHL) has 4 subcategories:
  - Lymphocyte-rich Hodgkin's lymphoma (LRHL), nodular sclerosing Hodgkin's lymphoma (NSHL), mixed cellularity Hodgkin's lymphoma (MCHL), and lymphocyte-depleted Hodgkin's lymphoma (LDHL)
  - NSHL is the most common subcategory
- » **Staging**
  - Ann Arbor staging system is most commonly used
  - Staged as A if there are no general symptoms
  - Staged as B if the patient experiences B symptoms
  - The diaphragm is used to divide stages
  - Stages 1 and 2: disease is above the diaphragm
  - Stages 3 and 4: disease is below the diaphragm
- » **Spread Patterns**
  - Spread occurs to adjacent lymph nodes
  - Spreads to the spleen in later stages
  - Can metastasize to liver, bone marrow, lungs and/or bone

- **Non-Hodgkin's lymphoma**
  - » Occurs anywhere in the body that lymph can travel (lymph nodes, organs, or a combination)
  - » Spreads randomly and in no order
  - » More common in older people, with 67 being the median age
  - » Exposure to ionizing radiation can cause lymphoma
  - » Common clinical presentations are swollen lymph nodes, night sweats, fatigue, itching, and weight loss (B symptoms)
  - » Common locations for NHL to occur are lymph nodes, GI tract (Peyer's patches), and Waldeyer's ring
  - » Chemotherapy used is CHOP (cyclophosphamide, vincristine, doxorubicin, and prednisone)
  - » **Pathology**
    - B-cell and T-cell neoplasms with 31 subtypes
    - Classified as follicular/nodular or diffuse
    - Diffuse lymphomas are more common
  - » **Staging**
    - Ann Arbor staging
    - Considers Waldeyer's ring, thymus, spleen, appendix, and Peyer's patches to be lymphatic tissues (not extralymphatic)
    - "X" indicates bulky disease
  - » **Spread Patterns**
    - Common nodal sites involved are the neck, groin, and axilla
    - Common extranodal spread is to the GI tract

9.. <u>Sarcomas (Bone and Soft Tissue)</u>
- **Anatomy**
  - » Soft tissue sarcomas (STS) occur in extraskeletal connective tissues that provide connection, support, and movement
  - » Common cells in the connective tissues are the mesoderm, primitive mesenchyme, and ectoderm
  - » Arise in structures that have connective tissues like blood vessel walls, pleura, pericardium, endothelium of blood vessels, bone, cartilage, muscles, and soft connective tissues
  - » Soft tissue sarcomas mostly occur in extremities in adults
  - » Soft tissue sarcomas mostly occur in the trunk, head, and neck for children
  - » Common symptoms are a painless, enlarging mass
  - » When irradiating sarcomas, it is important that the entire circumference of the extremity or area is not within the treatment field
    - A strip must be left so that lymph can be drained and to avoid edema

- **Lymphatics**
  - » Lymphatic spread is rare

- **Pathology**
  - » Sarcomas are named by the tissues they occur in
  - » 50 subtypes: leiomyosarcoma (smooth muscle), liposarcoma (fat), synovial sarcoma, malignant peripheral nerve sheath tumors, malignant fibrous histiocytomas (mixed fibroblasts and other cells)
  - » Most common in adults is malignant fibrous histiocytomas (MFH)
  - » Most common in children is rhabdomyosarcoma
  - » **Rhabdomyosarcoma**
    - Highly malignant tumors in the skeletal muscles that can occur in any location of the body
    - Examples: orbit, head and neck, parameningeal, genitourinary, extremity, trunk, retroperitoneum, etc.
  - » **Osteosarcoma**
    - Most common bone tumor
    - Occurs most frequently in the metaphysis of extremities like the distal femur or proximal tibia
    - Radioresistant
    - Peak age of diagnosis is 10 to 25
  - » **Ewing's sarcoma**
    - Second most common bone tumor
    - Occurs most frequently in the diaphysis of the femur
    - Has an onion-shaped appearance on radiographic images
    - Peak age of diagnosis is 10 to 20

» **Chondrosarcomas**
  - Bone tumors of the cartilage
  - Most commonly occurs in the pelvis
  - Occurs in the ribs, vertebrae, and long bones as well
  - Peak age of diagnosis is 35 to 60

- **Spread Patterns**
  » Aggressively spread to local areas
  » Most common site of distant spread is the lung
  » Less common sites of distant spread are the bones, liver and skin

10. Multiple Myeloma
- Malignancy of plasma cells
- Irregular absorption of bone that leads to painful boney lesions
- Occurs in the B-cell lymphocytes of the bone marrow
- Multiple lytic lesions
- The patient can be diagnosed when 10 percent of bone marrow cells are plasma cells upon aspiration
- Treated with radiation and chemotherapy

11. Skin
- **Anatomy**
  » Largest organ of the human body
  » Regulates body temperature and provides protection
  » Dermis = connective tissue layer
  » Epidermis = epithelial layer
    - Has two layers: outermost is the stratum corneum and the basal layer (separates epidermis from dermis)
  » Melanocytes = cells that produce the skin's pigment
    - Located between basal cells within the epidermis

- **Lymphatics**
  » Lymph nodes involved depend on location of skin cancer

- **Pathology: Non-Melanomas**
  » **Basal cell carcinoma (BCC)**
    - Skin cancer in the stem cells of the deepest layer of the skin (stratum basale)
    - Slow-growing and unlikely to metastasize
    - Most common type of skin cancer
    - Four subtypes: nodular-ulcerated BCC, superficial BCC, morpheaform/sclerosing BCC, and cystic BCC

- » **Squamous cell carcinoma**
  - • Skin cancer in the superficial layers of the epidermis
  - • Grows faster than BCC and has an increased chance of metastasis
  - • Can appear anywhere on the body but is most common on areas that have been exposed to the sun like the head, neck, face, arms, and hands
- » Other histopathologic types: adenocarcinomas, cutaneous T-cell lymphoma, Kaposi sarcoma, and Merkel cell carcinoma

- **Pathology: Melanoma**
  - » Most aggressive skin cancer
  - » Most occur from a change in a nevus that already existed
  - » Arise from melanocytes in the basal layer of the epidermis
  - » ABCD rule can help detect melanomas:
    - • Asymmetry: melanomas are typically not symmetrical
    - • Border: melanomas have irregular and uneven borders
    - • Color: melanomas are not uniform and have various shades of black or brown
    - • Diameter: melanomas typically have a diameter larger than 6 mm
  - » Changes in the mole can signify melanomas as well
    - • Change in color, surface, texture, or skin around the mole
  - » Melanoma categories: superficial spreading melanomas (SSMs), nodular melanomas (NMs), lentigo maligna melanomas (LMMs) and acral lentiginous melanomas (ALMs)
  - » Common locations for melanomas are on the face and scalp

- **Spread patterns**
  - » Skin cancers mainly spread through direct extension
  - » Melanomas can have satellite metastasis around the primary tumor
  - » Melanomas can spread to any organ
  - » Melanomas first spread by direct extension, then to regional lymph nodes, then to distant organs such as the liver, bone, or brain
  - » Non-melanomas can metastasize to the liver, bone, brain, or lung

12. Leukemia
- • Leukemia develops during the formation of blood and lymphocytes
- • Pluripotent stem cells form into erythrocytes, neutrophils, eosinophils, basophils, monocytes, platelets, or lymphocytes
- • With leukemia, hematopoietic or lymphopoietic production is uncontrolled and accelerated
  - » Cells can be defective
  - » Cells' maturation may be incomplete
- • Leukemic cells build up in the bone marrow, which can affect the production of red blood cells, white blood cells, and platelets
- • **Staging** = FAB (French, American, British)
- • Common treatment is bone marrow transplants, which require total body irradiation (TBI)

- **ALL (Acute Lymphocytic Leukemia)**
  - » Overgrowth of lymphoblasts, which limits the growth of healthy cells
  - » Symptoms appear from this limitation of normal healthy cells
  - » 50 percent of all leukemias are acute leukemias
  - » Most common pediatric disease
  - » Mostly occurs in children ages 2 to 3 and doesn't commonly occur past the age of 15
  - » Possible correlation to radiation from atomic bomb explosions or nuclear accidents
  - » Treated with radiation therapy, chemotherapy, and bone marrow transplants

- **AML (Acute Myelogenous Leukemia)**
  - » Overgrowth of cells that are unable to differentiate in response to hormonal signals and cellular interactions
  - » Do not mature or mature with defects
  - » 80 percent of adults who have acute leukemia have AML
  - » Patients are usually older than 40 (median age is 67)
  - » Diagnosed because Auer rods are present in leukemic cells
  - » Treated with radiation therapy, chemotherapy, and bone marrow transplants

- **CLL (Chronic Lymphocytic Leukemia)**
  - » Increased amount of leukemic cells in the bone marrow, blood, lymph nodes, and spleen
    - Organs become enlarged
    - Bone marrow function is lessened
  - » 30 percent of all leukemias
  - » Risk of developing CLL increases with age (average age is 65)
  - » Exposure to radiation is not a risk factor
  - » Heredity may be a risk factor
  - » Possible treatments are chemotherapy, radiation therapy, and surgery

- **CML (Chronic Myelogenous Leukemia)**
  - » Abnormal hematopoietic stem cells that contain the Philadelphia chromosome
  - » Increase in granulocytes and megakaryocytes
  - » Erythrocytes become damaged
  - » 15 percent of all adult types of leukemias
  - » Rare in children; common age is mid-60s
  - » Three stages: chronic, accelerated, and blast crisis
  - » Treated with radiation therapy, chemotherapy, and bone marrow transplants

13. Mycosis Fungoides
   - Subgroup of cutaneous T-cell lymphoma
   - Lesions occur anywhere on the body, but are most common in areas that are exposed to the sun
   - Three phases: patch/premycotic phase, infiltrated plaque/mycotic phase, and tumor/fungoid phase
   - Can invade lymph nodes, spleen, lungs, liver, and bone marrow
   - Malignant T-cells
   - Treated with radiation and chemotherapy
      » Total-skin electron beam (TSEB) therapy is a treatment option
      » Topical chemotherapy can be used
      » Systemic chemotherapy is used when the disease becomes widespread

14. Bone Marrow Transplant (BMT)
   - Treatment for ALL, AML, and CML
   - Healthy bone marrow is taken from an appropriate donor and is then introduced into the patient who has diseased bone marrow that has been destroyed by chemotherapy or total body irradiation (TBI)
   - The best donors are identical twins
   - Autologous BMT: the patient's own bone marrow is reinfused after leukemic cells have been removed
   - Allogeneic BMT: bone marrow is donated by a compatible donor
   - Syngeneic BMT: bone marrow is donated by an identical twin
   - Examples of BMT failures are reoccurrence or graft-versus-host disease

15. Benign Diseases
   - **Heterotopic bone**
      » Heterotopic ossification happens in some patients who undergo hip surgery
      » Bone forms in the soft tissue, where bone does not typically form
      » Treatment occurs preoperatively or postoperatively
      » Treatment is one dose of about 6 to 8 Gy

   - **Keloid**
      » Unwarranted amount of scar formation
      » Benign condition of uncontrolled growth of connective tissue
      » Controlled with surgery and low-dose radiation afterward
         - Radiation treatment should occur within 24 hours of surgery
      » Typically treated in three fractions to a total of 900 to 1,500 cGy

- **Arteriovenous Malformations (AVM)**
  - » An abnormality where the arteries and veins become tangled and are unable to transfer nutrients to vital organs, such as the brain
  - » Complications of AVMs are seizures and hemorrhaging
  - » Treated with surgery or radiosurgery
  - » Commonly treated with doses of 1,200 to 2,500 cGy

16. Emergencies In Oncology
  - In certain cases, patients may require emergency doses of radiation
  - Oncologic emergencies are indicated for tumors pressing on and obstructing the superior vena cava, skeletal metastasis, brain metastasis that cause increased intracranial pressure, and vaginal bleeding
  - In these cases, it is common to give one or two treatments with high doses to reduce the symptoms
    - » Treatment fields are typically simple open fields with no field shaping
  - After these initial treatments, the doses are lessened to average treatment doses with a treatment plan using MLCs and other field shaping
  - These treatments are typically palliative

B. Determining the Type of Tumor
1. Histopathology
  - **Benign** tumors are those that do not spread or metastasize and closely resemble the tissue of origin
    - » Benign tumors usually do not grow fast and are encapsulated
  - **Malignant** tumors have the ability to spread or metastasize and do not closely resemble the cells of their origin (anaplastic)
    - » Malignant tumors grow rapidly and are life threatening
  - **Carcinomas** are malignant tumors that occur in epithelial tissues
    - » Most common tumors
    - » Spread through the lymphatic system
    - » Example: squamous cell, adenocarcinomas
  - **Sarcomas** are malignant tumors that do not occur in epithelial tissues
    - » Typical areas are bone, connective tissues, or soft tissue
    - » Spread through the bloodstream

2. <u>Grade</u>
   a. Use of Grading System
   - The grade explains how aggressive a tumor is
   - The more aggressive a tumor is, the higher the grade
   - The less aggressive a tumor is, the lower the grade

   b. Details of Grading System
   - The grading system is an example of how differentiated the tumor is (or how well it resembles the normal tissue of origin)
   - Graded in numbers 1 to 4
     » Lower numbers are assigned to tumors that are well differentiated and are less likely to metastasize
     » Higher numbers are assigned to tumors that are less differentiated, are more advanced, and can easily metastasize
   - "GX" means that the grade is not determined

3. <u>Stage</u>
   a. Use of Staging System
   - Staging explains the size and depth of the tumor
   - Can be staged clinically or pathologically, or a combination of the two

   b. Details of Staging System
   - TNM staging depicts the extent of the tumor using three subgroups
     » T = size of the primary tumor and if it has invaded areas
     » N = involvement of regional lymph nodes
     » M = presence of metastatic disease
     » Each subgroup can be assigned a numerical subscript to show the extent of the subgroup
     » "X" is assigned if the subgroup is unable to be determined
   - There are two key staging systems: American Joint Committee on Cancer (AJCC system) and Union for International Cancer Control (UICC system)
   - FIGO staging is used for gynecological cancers
   - Dukes staging is used for colorectal tumors
   - Ann Arbor staging is used for lymphatic staging
     » "A" or "B" describes the if the patient is lacking or has "B" symptoms

Part 2: Dosimetry

A. Various Treatment Types and Procedures

1. Different Types of Radiation Therapy Treatments

- **3-D Conformal Radiation Therapy:** conforms the radiation beam so that the target volume receives the prescribed dose and the surrounding healthy tissue receives a much lower dose
  - » Planned using 3-D imaging, such as computed tomography
- **Electron Beam:** a monoenergetic beam that is used for superficial tumors
  - » Scatters easily and needs a cone to confine the beam
  - » Field edges balloon out because of scatter and aren't definitive like photon beams
  - » There is a "rapid falloff" of dose, which means that deeper organs and tissues will receive very little or no dose
- **IMRT:** "Intensity-Modulated Radiation Therapy"
  - » A radiation beam that has varying intensities throughout the beam
    - Many smaller beams or "beamlets"
    - Beamlets are commonly as small as 1 cm x 1 cm
  - » The dose is not uniform
  - » Allows for higher doses to tumors while minimizing doses to surrounding healthy tissues
  - » Uses inverse treatment planning and dynamic MLCs
- **Stereotactic Radiosurgery (SRS):** treats small tumors within the cranium at a high dose
  - » Treats tumors with only one fraction
  - » Tumors are usually less than 3 cm
  - » Treatment positioning must be accurate within ± 1 mm
  - » SRS of intracranial lesions may require a frame attached to the patient's head
  - » Common diseases SRS treats within the cranium:
    - Arteriovenous malformations (AVMs)
    - Trigeminal neuralgia
    - Acoustic neuromas
    - Meningiomas
    - Pituitary adenomas
    - Metastatic and primary brain tumors
  - » SRS can also treat some tumors within the spine (less common)
  - » Examples of machines that can perform SRS are Gamma Knife and CyberKnife
- **Stereotactic Body Radiation Therapy:** treats small tumors outside of the cranium with a very high dose for about 3 to 5 fractions
- **Total-Body Irradiation:** radiation therapy that targets the whole body to prepare for bone marrow transplants and to treat other malignancies
- **IGRT:** "Image-Guided Radiotherapy"
  - » Patient is imaged prior to treatment to confirm the position
  - » Shifts of the table position can be made before treatment for more accuracy in treatment delivery
  - » Examples: EPID, KV and MV cone-beam CT, and ultrasound

- **Particle Beam Radiotherapy:** high-energy charged particles, such as protons, alpha particles, and carbon ions
  - » The dose curve of a proton beam starts off low at the beginning, but then rapidly rises toward the end of the path and then abruptly falls to zero (Bragg peak)

2. <u>Cross Sectional CT Images and Anatomy</u>

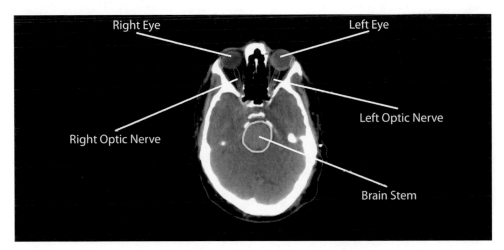

Axial view of the brain and orbits

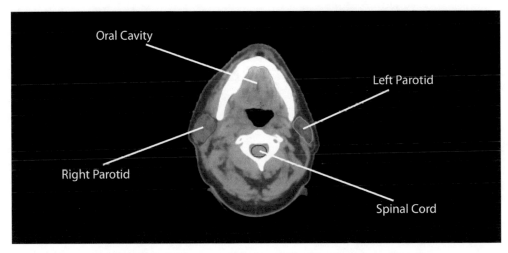

Axial view of the parotid glands in the head and neck

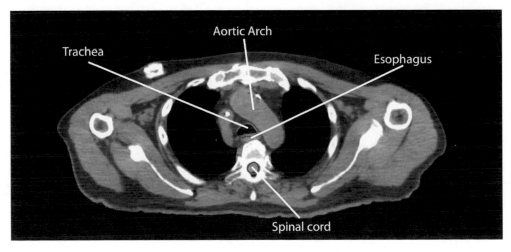

Axial view of the superior portion of the lungs

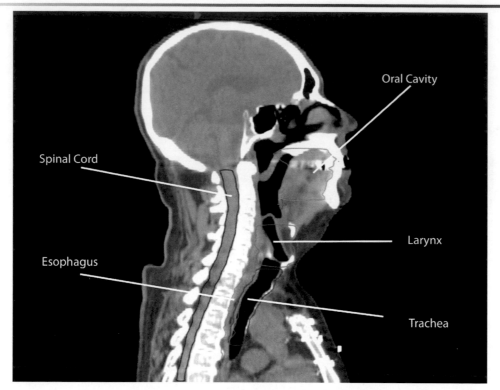

Sagittal view of the head and neck

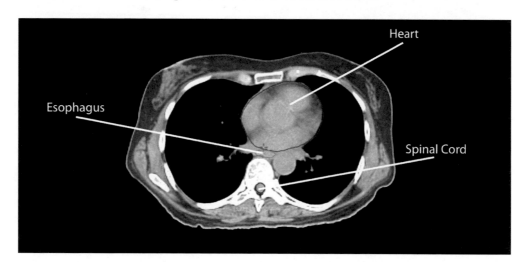

Axial view of the heart and lungs

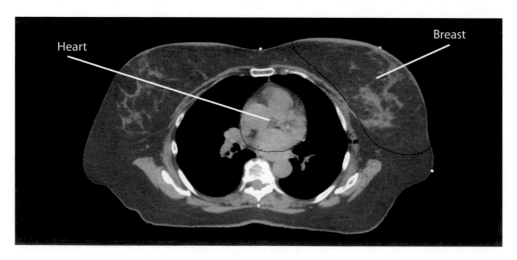

Axial view of the breast and heart

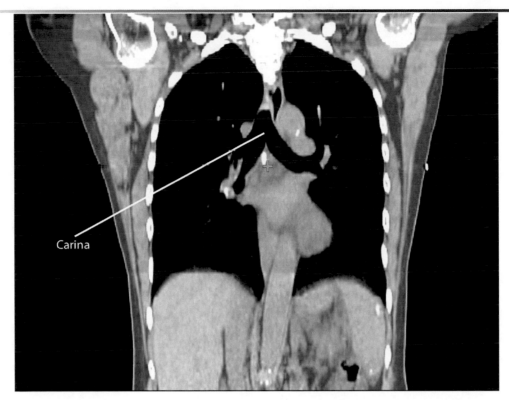

Coronal view of the lungs

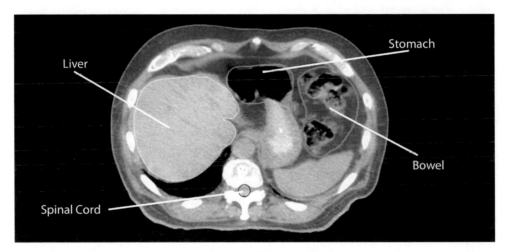

Axial view of the abdomen

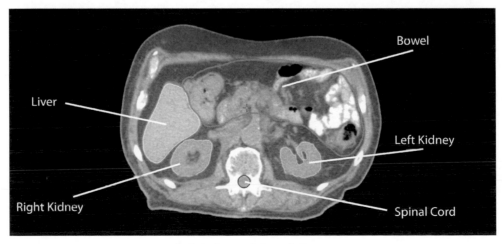

Axial view of the abdomen

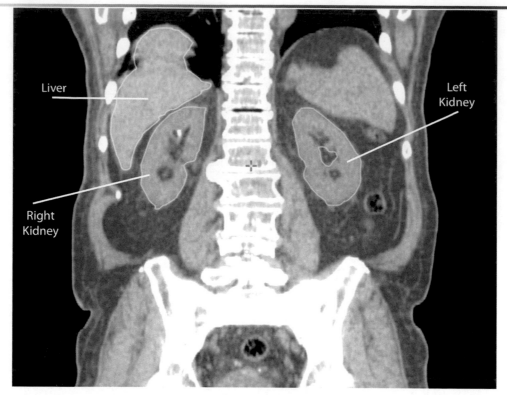

Coronal view of the abdomen

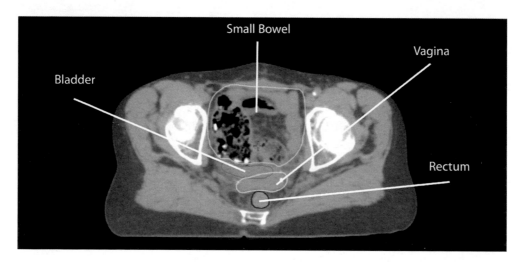

Axial view of the female pelvis

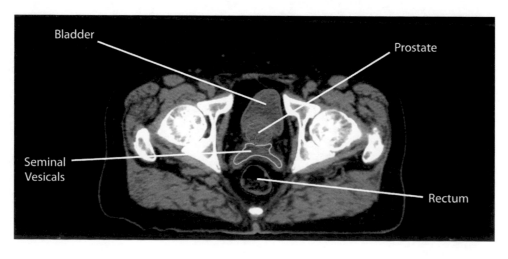

Axial view of the male pelvis

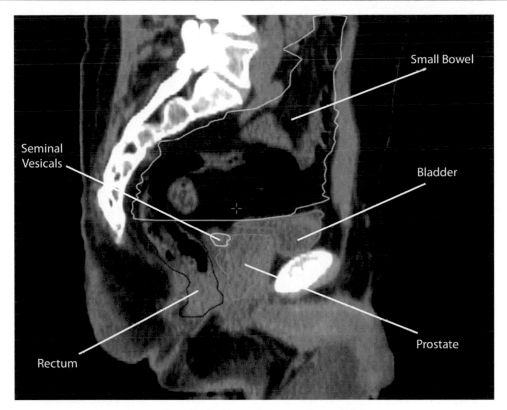

Sagittal view of the male pelvis

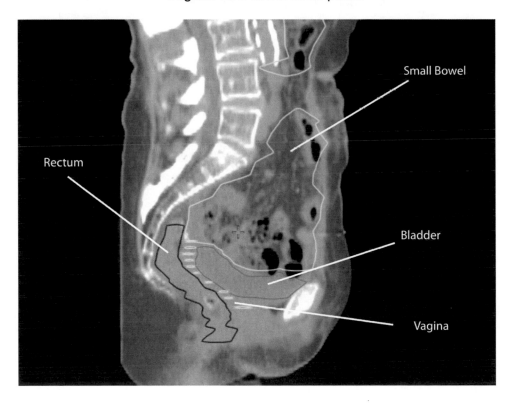

Sagittal view of the female pelvis

3. Immobilization Techniques
- Common patient positions are supine and prone
- Patient setup must be reproducible from the CT simulation to each daily treatment
- The patient is lined up using lasers mounted on the walls and ceilings and the tattoo marks on the patient's skin
- **Patient positioning aids:** help to position patient for treatment
  - » Does not limit the patient's movement
  - » Can be used for multiple patients
  - » Examples: head holders, sponge pillows, foam cushions, neck rolls
- **Complex immobilization devices:** limit the patient's movement and create a very reproducible patient setup
  - » Customized for each patient
  - » Examples: Alpha Cradle, Vac-Lok, thermoplastic molds, bite blocks
- **Simple immobilization devices:** help to constrain patient
  - » Used with positioning aids
  - » Not as restricting as complex immobilization devices
  - » Examples: tape, rubber band, arm-to-foot straps

4. Contrast Media
- Contrast media is often used during the simulation process
- The contrast will highlight specific organs to further help create the treatment plan
  - » Contrast can highlight the area to be treated
  - » Contrast can highlight critical structures to be avoided

B. CT Simulation
1. Components
- Computed tomography is the most common imaging modality used for radiation therapy treatment planning
- Images are produced by using x-ray, detectors, and a computer
- Computed tomography CT is spiral, or helical, which means the couch moves as the x-ray tube rotates within the gantry
- Milliamperage (mA) measures the beam quantity, or how many x-rays are produced
  - » An increase in mA leads to a higher patient dose
  - » Tube current is measured in coulomb/sec
- Slice thickness and space between slices are key factors for generating high-quality digitally reconstructed radiographs (DRRs)
  - » Spacing should be lower than 5 mm
  - » Slice thickness is typically 2 to 3 mm

2. <u>Imaging Terminology</u>
- **Field of view (FOV):** the diameter of the area being scanned
- **Scan field of view:** area of interest to be scanned
- **Window width (WW):** the number of shades of gray displayed on an image or the contrast of the image
  - » A narrow window width has more contrast
- **Window level (WL):** the median shade of gray or Hounsfield unit within the window width
  - » Changes image brightness
  - » An increase of window level creates a darker image
  - » A decrease of window level creates a brighter image
- **CT number:** a value that represents a shade of gray, also known as the Hounsfield unit
  - » Represents the density of different tissues (electron density)
  - » The numbers range from -1,000 to +1,000
    - -1,000 represents air
    - 0 represents water
    - +1,000 represents bone
- **Reconstruction:** the computer uses algorithms to create the CT image in different planes
  - » Coronal and sagittal views are reconstructed from axial slices
  - » Digitally reconstructed radiographs (DDRs) look like plain radiographs and are reconstructed from the CT slices to show a beam's-eye view
    - Made to be able to compare to portal films

3. <u>Useful Information For Treatment Planning</u>
- A contour is a 3-D image taken in the treatment position that provides data of the anatomy of the patient, such as the skin, tumor, and other organs within the body
- A contour is a representation of the patient and is necessary for creating accurate treatment plans and calculating doses
- Target volumes, critical structures, and other anatomy are defined on the CT, MRI and/or PET images
- In the virtual simulator, the physician can identify the treatment borders and the isocenter location
- Multiple studies from different imaging modalities can be fused together to give even more information to those planning the treatments
- It is common to fuse together MRI and CT images
- MRI scans are useful to show soft tissues
  - » MRI and CT scans are commonly fused together to better highlight and define the prostate
- PET scans are useful because they show the activity of the tumor
  - » PET and CT scans are commonly fused together to show areas of activity in sites such as the lung, and head and neck
- There are two different ways to plan a treatment once all the data is gathered, known as forward and inverse planning

- **Forward planning:** the planner chooses the energy, number, shape, and direction of the radiation beams
    - » The computer calculates the isodose lines, and the planner must assess the dose distribution and make changes if necessary
- **Inverse planning:** the planner chooses the energy, appropriate dose to the tumor, and the tolerances of the normal healthy tissues
    - » The computer then creates a plan with beam MLC patterns, shapes, directions, etc.
    - » Used in IMRT (Intensity-Modulated Radiation Therapy)

4. Transferring and Storing Images
- Images can be transmitted via magnetic tapes, optical disks, or an electronic network
- **DICOM (Digital Imaging and Communications in Medicine)** creates the standard format to transfer images from imaging computers to the treatment planning computer
- **Picture Archiving and Communication System (PACS)** is used to store and share images electronically

5. Lasers
- Lasers are used to mark the patient in three areas to be able to triangulate and position the patient in a reproducible position for daily treatments
- Within treatment and simulation rooms, lasers are located laterally, sagittally, and overhead on the ceiling in the X, Y, and Z coordinates

C. Recording Simulation Factors In Patient Charts
1. Patient Position
- The patient's anatomic position is determined at the time of the simulation
- Descriptions such as supine, prone, head first, feet first, arms up, arms down, etc., are important to document so that the patient's position is reproducible

2. Devices
- Equipment such as the patient's immobilization should be clearly written as well
    - » Examples: neck roll used, positioning sponges, wing boards, breast boards, prone belly boards, etc.
- Equipment such as the gantry angle will be determined during treatment planning
    - » This information can be found in the treatment plan and should be compared with the patient's actual setup
- Accessories used for treatment (such as wedges, blocks, or bolus) will also be located within the treatment plan

3. Visual Aids For Setup
- Photographs of patient's position should be taken and added to the patient's chart so that the therapist who is setting up the patient can reproduce the setup created at the time of the simulation
- Pictures or diagrams showing the locations of the tattoos should also be included in the patient's chart as a reference to make sure the therapist sets up to the appropriate marks

Part 3: Treatment Dose and Prescription

A. Prescription

1. Total Dose

- Total doses change depending on the location of the tumor and the organs at risk surrounding the tumor
- An example of typical curative doses are daily fractions of 180 to 200 cGy to a total dose of 5,400-6,000 cGy
- An example of a typical palliative dose is a daily fraction of 300 cGy to a total dose of 3,000 cGy
- A boost or a cone-down field is a smaller field that can give a higher dose

2. Fractionation

- Common fraction schedules are once a day, five days a week, for several weeks
- The amount of fractions varies with the total tumor dose
- "BID" means to treat twice a day
    - » There must be six hours between fractions

3. Beam Energy

- The beam energy used for treatments is chosen depending on the thickness of the patient and the depth of the tumor
- Tumors in areas of the body that are thicker use higher beam energies
    - » For example: most treatments for pelvic tumors use 15x
- Tumors in areas of the body that aren't as thick use lower beam energies
    - » For example: most treatments for brain tumors use 6x
- Different beam energies have different depths for d_{max}

4. Radiation Type

- **Alpha particles:** two protons and two neutrons, also known as a helium nuclei, released from an unstable heavy nuclei as it decays
    - » Has a charge, a heavy mass, and a high LET
    - » Travels short distances but creates a lot of damage in that distance
    - » Common in atomic numbers greater than 82
- **Beta particles:** electrons released by the nucleus
    - » Negatively charged (negatron) or positively charged (positron)
    - » Travel farther and penetrate farther than alpha particles
- **X-rays:** electromagnetic radiation, known as photons
    - » No mass and no charge
    - » Manmade
    - » Interaction occurs near the nucleus
- **Gamma rays:** photons naturally emitted from a nucleus
    - » Gamma rays and x-rays penetrate farther than alpha particles and beta particles
- **Natural background radiation:** cosmic rays, terrestrial radiation, and radionuclides in the human body

5. Treatment Volume
- **Gross tumor volume (GTV)** is the tumor volume that is visible or can be palpated
- **Clinical target volume (CTV)** is the GTV and the area around it that may have microscopic disease
- **Planning target volume (PTV)** is the CTV and an area around it to give a margin for uncertainties
    » Examples of uncertainties: patient motion, penumbra, variations of treatment setup
- **Internal target volume (ITV)** accounts for the CTV plus motion of the tumor caused by breathing or involuntary motions
- **Treated volume** is the area that is contained within the isodose curve
- **Irradiated volume** is the volume of tissues that is given a large portion of the dose
- **Organs at risk (OAR)** are organs close to the irradiated area that may effect or limit the dosage delivered

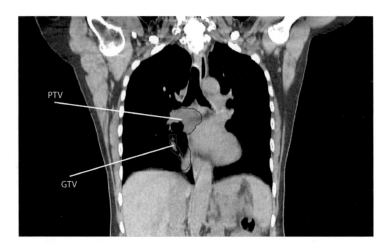

6. Treatment Fields and Techniques
- Treatment fields are established based on tolerance doses of the organs at risk and the dose distributions
- Field orientation is arranged depending on the location and organs at risk near the tumor
- MLCs and other beam modifiers can be used to further shape the beam
- Adequate dose distributions usually require multiple fields
- Single fields are usually used for a posterior spine field
- Parallel opposed portal (POP) has a hinge angle of 180 degrees
    » Example: AP and PA fields
    » Example: left lateral and right lateral fields
- Three-field technique is commonly used for structures within the abdomen, such as the pancreas, bladder, rectum, etc.
- Four-field technique/four-field box is commonly used for deep tumors within the pelvis or abdomen
    » Fields are 90 degrees apart from each other
- Wedge-pair technique has a hinge angle that is less than 180 degrees between two fields
    » Requires wedges to have a more even dose distribution
    » The thick ends of the wedges, also known as the "heel," face each other
    » Commonly used for more superficial tumors

7. Rotational Fields
- Rotational fields are also known as "arc therapy," where the radiation is delivered while the gantry is moving in an arc from one set point to another
- For arcs less than 360 degrees, the treatment planning method is called **past pointing**
  - » The treatment plans for the beam to treat to a depth farther than the center of the tumor
- For arcs that are 360 degrees, the beam is set to treat at the exact depth of the center of the tumor
- Arc speed is calculated as MU/degree
- Before treating with an arc, the therapist should do a dry run of the gantry rotation to ensure there will be no collisions between the gantry and the patient or table

8. Fixed Fields
- For fixed fields, the gantry does not move while the radiation beam is delivered
  - » The gantry moves between each field while the beam is off
  - » The gantry is stationary while the beam is being delivered

9. Field Weighting
- Doses from multiple fields are not always equal
- Usually used when the tumor does not lie at mid-depth or when one beam may be going through a critical structure
- Beam angles can contribute different doses toward the total dose
  - » Example: AP:PA weighted 2:1 respectively
    - The AP field will deliver 2/3 of the dose
    - Multiply the total prescription dose by 2/3 to find the amount of cGy delivered in the AP field
    - The PA field will deliver 1/3 of the dose
    - Multiply the total prescription dose by 1/3 to find the amount of cGy delivered in the PA field

10. Treatment Machine Properties
- Isocenter = 100 cm
- Max field size = 40x40 cm @ 100 SSD
- Photon therapy energies range from about 4 to 35 MV
- Electron therapy energies range from about 4 to 22 MeV
- Treatment table can hold up to 350 pounds

11. Changes In Treatment Plans
- Any changes in the plan must be recognized prior to the patient's next treatment
- If the changes include the field size or shape, the new field must be imaged for confirmation
- Changes in fractionation or dose must be properly documented and followed as prescribed

12. Beam Modifiers
- **Bolus** is placed between the radiation source and the patient's skin
  - » It brings the dose closer to the skin's surface and decreases skin sparing
  - » Bolus will attenuate some of the beam
- **Wedges** and **compensators** are used to alter the isodose distribution based on the patient's skin contour
  - » Compensators are made of a high-density material, like Cerrobend or "poly lead"
  - » Compensators are rarely used now and have been replaced by IMRT
  - » Wedges are also made of a high-density material, like lead or steel
  - » Newer machines use enhanced dynamic wedges (EDW) to replace the use of physical wedges
  - » Instead of a physical wedge that is placed into the treatment head, an EDW uses the motion of the Y-jaw to mimic a wedge
    - • EDWs change the isodose distribution just like wedges
    - • Planned in the treatment planning process
- A **beam spoiler** is used in larger fields like Total Body Irradiation (TBI) and eliminates skin sparing
  - » Solid plastic tray
  - » Increases dose to skin without decreasing the penetration of the beam

B. Treatment Planning Parameters
1. Field Size
- Measurements of the treatment field are defined at the isocenter (width x length)
- The field size is created by two pairs of the secondary asymmetric collimator jaws
- Fields can be further shaped using MLCs and/or custom Cerrobend blocks
- DRRs are a document of the field parameters
- The physical radiation field size is delineated at the 50 percent isodose line

2. Tumor Depth
- Tumor depth is established with 3-D imaging
- Depth of the tumor determines the energy of the beam and the type of treatment
- Superficial tumors are most likely to be treated with electrons
- Deeper tumors are most likely to be treated with photons

3. Patient Separation
- Other terms are patient thickness, intrafield distance, and innerfield distance (IFD)
- Measured at the central axis and at specific points within the treatment field
- Can be measured with a caliper, which is a ruler with one sliding leg and one stationary leg

4. SSD

- **SSD** = source-to-surface distance
  - » Distance from the source of radiation to the patient's skin surface
  - » If using an isocentric or SAD technique, the SSD will change at different gantry angles
  - » For SSD techniques, the SSD is 100 cm or another specified "fixed" SSD
    - Patient may need to be moved between fields
    - More chance of an error
  - » Used for single fields or to be able to obtain larger field sizes
  - » Used for electron fields

5. SAD

- **SAD** = source-to-axis distance
  - » Distance from the source of radiation to the isocenter
  - » In current linear accelerators, the SAD is 100 cm
  - » In older Cobalt-60 machines, the SAD was 80 cm
  - » "Isocentric technique" is when the isocenter is located within the patient
    - The SSD is less than 100 cm
    - Patient doesn't need to be moved in between fields
    - Less chance of errors in treatment

6. Collimator Parameters

- The secondary collimating jaws are moveable and asymmetric
- These jaws can create rectangular field sizes ranging from 0x0 cm to 40x40 cm at the isocenter
- Jaws are made of tungsten
- Only <0.5 percent transmission through the jaws is permitted
- As field size increases, collimator scatter is increased
  - » Collimator scatter contributes to dose, therefore less MU is needed

7. Abutting Fields

- Abutting or adjacent fields meet at a determined depth within the patient because of beam divergence
- To avoid hot spots or cold spots, there must be a gap on the skin surface
- Gap calculation:
  $$S = \tfrac{1}{2} L_1(d/SSD) + \tfrac{1}{2} L_2(d/SSD) \quad \text{or} \quad S = d/2(L_1/SSD + L_2/SSD)$$
  - » L = field length
  - » d = depth
  - » SSD = source-to-surface distance
- Commonly used in craniospinal irradiation (CSI)
  - » Orthogonal field areas of possible overlap: laterals for the cranium and PA fields for the spine
  - » Beam divergence causes overlap between the cranium and spine fields and between the multiple spine fields
  - » It is especially important to avoid overlap and hot spots of the spinal cord

» Other techniques to avoid overlap are half-beam block, beam splitters, or couch rotation

» Calculation of the couch angle to avoid overlap:

Arc tan Ø = (½ field width/SAD)

• "Feathering" is a technique used to move or change the location of the gap throughout the treatment

» Adjusted at least two or three times during the entire treatment after so many fractions

» Usually, the gap location is changed every five fractions

» Blurs any inhomogeneous doses within the gap area

» The central axis remains the same, but the field lengths change

8. Image Fusion

• Image fusion uses multiple imaging modalities to provide better visualization of the patient's anatomy

• The images from different modalities are fused or laid over one another to create a more informative image

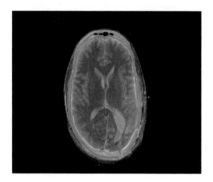

MRI fused with CT scan

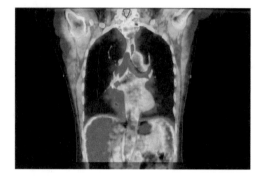

PET scan fused with CT scan

C. Dose Calculation

1. Beam Energy

• The beam energy that is used for treatment is determined by the depth of the tumor and the separation of the patient in the area of the tumor

• Photon beams are more penetrating than electron beams

» The percentage depth dose at the patient's skin surface is around 30 percent for photon beams

• Electron beams are used more for superficial tumors; the percentage depth dose at the patient's skin surface is around 80 to 90 percent

• Treatments using electrons are usually prescribed to the 80 to 90 percent isodose line

• As a general rule for electron beams, MeV is about three times the max depth of the tumor

• To determine isodose lines for electrons (E = energy for electron beam):

» E/2 = 50 percent isodose line (useful range of electrons)

» E/3 = 80 percent isodose line

» E/4 = 90 percent isodose line (therapeutic range of electrons)

2. Calculating The Equivalent Square

- For dosimetric calculations, all rectangular treatment fields must be converted to squares
- To determine the equivalent square from the rectangular open field, use the following equations:

    EqSq = (2ab)/(a+b) or (4 x area)/perimeter
    - » a = length of one side of rectangle
    - » b = length of other side of rectangle (perpendicular to "a")
- Equivalent square values can also be found on lookup tables
- Blocked fields are fields that use MLCs or blocks to change the shape of the treatment field
- To determine the equivalent square of a blocked field, use the following equation:

    $f'd \approx f_d \sqrt{1\text{-}a}$
    - » f_d = unblocked field
    - » a = fraction of the field that is blocked
    - » Unblocked field times the square root of 1 minus the fraction of the area blocked
    - » Or the square root of the open area minus the blocked area
    - » Example: the open area is 20x10 and the blocked area is 4x6
        - First do the equation (20x10) – (4x6), then take the square root of the answer
- Clarkson integration can be used to find the area of irregularly shaped fields
    - » Uses multiple "pie-shaped" sections to re-create the shape of the field
    - » Takes scatter from the blocked area into consideration for calculations

3. Scatter Factors

- The main cause of collimator scatter is from photons scattering within the head of the gantry
    - » Mostly occurs with the flattening filter
    - » Bigger field sizes create more scatter
    - » Smaller field sizes create less scatter
- Scatter that happens within the patient or phantom is called phantom scatter
    - » Amount of scatter depends on the volume of tissue within the treatment field
    - » As the field size increases, the amount of phantom scatter increases
    - » Cannot be directly measured
- Collimator and phantom scatter factors are located on lookup tables
- Backscatter factor (BSF) and peak scatter factor (PSF) both compare the dose rate in free space to the dose rate within a phantom at the d_{max}
    - » Backscatter factor (BSF) is used for low-energy beams
    - » Peak scatter factor (PSF) is used for high-energy beams
        - Beams above 4MV

4. D$_{max}$

- D$_{max}$ is the depth where electronic equilibrium is reached and 100 percent of the dose is delivered
    - » The amount of energy lost is equivalent to the amount of energy gained
- The d$_{max}$ for higher-energy beams is deeper
    - » As energy is increased, skin sparing is also increased for photon beams

Energy	D$_{max}$
4 MV	1 cm
6 MV	1.5 cm
10 MV	2.5 cm
15 MV	3.0 cm
18 MV	3.2 cm
20 MV	3.5 cm
25 MV	5.0 cm
6 MeV	1.5 cm
9 MeV	2.2 cm
12 MeV	2.8 cm
Co-60	0.5 cm

5. Percentage Depth Dose (PDD)

- A ratio that compares the absorbed dose at a depth to the absorbed dose at a specific reference dose (d$_{max}$)
    - » Stated as a percentage
    - » PDD = (absorbed dose at depth)/(absorbed dose at d$_{max}$) x 100 percent
- Only used to calculate MU in SSD treatments (not SAD treatments)
- PDD changes depending on four components: energy, depth, field size, and SSD
    - » An increase of energy, field size, and SSD cause an increase in PDD
        - Direct relationship
        - The higher the energy, the more penetrating the beam, so a higher percentage of dose is present at a specific depth compared with low-energy beams
        - An increase of field size causes an increase of PDD because there is more scatter, which contributes to the dose
        - Field size is measured on the skin's surface
        - PDD increases as the distance from the source of radiation to the patient increases as the beam builds up before reaching d$_{max}$
    - » As the depth within the patient increases past d$_{max}$, the PDD decreases
        - Inverse relationship
        - The radiation beam is attenuated as it travels through the patient, so less of the beam is present at greater depths
- To determine the increase in PDD when there is a change in SSD, use the following equation to determine the Mayneord F Factor:
    - » $[(SSD_2 + d_{max})/(SSD_1 + d_{max})]^2 \times [(SSD_1 + depth)/(SSD_2 + depth)]^2$
    - » The Mayneord F Factor makes up for the change in dose at different depths of the central axis due to the inverse square law

6. TAR

- Tissue air ratio (TAR) is the ratio of an absorbed dose at a depth within the phantom at a given distance compared with the absorbed dose in free space at the same distance
- TAR is independent of SSD
- Dependent on energy, field size, and depth
    - » As the energy increases, the beam becomes more penetrating and TAR increases
    - » Increasing the field size causes an increase in TAR because there is more scatter adding to the dose
    - » TAR decreases as depth increases past d_{max} due to beam attenuation

7. TMR

- Tissue maximum ratio (TMR) is the ratio of an absorbed dose at a specified depth in a phantom to the absorbed dose at d_{max} at the same distance from the radiation source
    - » TMR = (dose in tissue)/(dose in phantom d_{max})
    - » Distance from the source does not change, but the amount of material/tissue between the depth and source may change
- TMR is used to measure doses of high-energy beams
- The value of TMR is usually less than 1.0
- Used to calculate MU in SAD, or isocentric, setups

8. SSD

- When calculating MU for SSD techniques, percent depth dose (PDD) is used in the equation
    - » Doses are calculated to d_{max} or when PDD is equal to 100 percent

9. SAD

- When calculating MU for SAD techniques, tissue maximum ratio (TMR) is used in the equation
- Most machines are typically calibrated to deliver 1 cGy per MU for a 10x10 field size at a depth of d_{max}
    - » However, machines can be calibrated to 100 SSD or 100 SAD

10. Inverse Square Calculations

- Describes the correlation between the distance from the source of radiation and the intensity of the beam
- The intensity of the radiation beam is inversely proportionate to the square of the distance from the source of radiation
- Equation of the inverse square law:
    $$I_1/I_2 = (D_2 / D_1)^2$$
    - » I = intensity
    - » D = distance
- This can be explained by beam divergence
- When the distance is increased, the same amount of radiation spreads to a larger area and the intensity is reduced

- Example: if the distance is increased by two, the intensity of the beam is decreased by one fourth of the original amount
- Example: if the distance is decreased by two, the intensity is increased by four times the original amount

11. <u>Extended Distance Factors</u>
- Extended distances have SSDs that are greater than the isocenter (100 cm)
- Extended distances are necessary when larger field sizes are required
  - » Examples: total body irradiation, total skin irradiation, and some mantle fields
    - TBI has an SSD of several meters
- When SSDs are changed and extended, the change of PDD (percentage depth dose) is calculated by using the Mayneord F Factor
- The Mayneord F Factor uses the principles of inverse square law
- Needed to calculate MU for extended distances

12. <u>Wedges</u>
- Wedges change the shape of the isodose curve
- To find the desired wedge angle, use the following calculation:
    Wedge angle = 90 − (hinge angle/2)
- Higher wedge angles create a steeper isodose curve
- Isodose lines for wedged fields are less steep at greater depths due to scatter
- The angle of the wedge is not determined by the angle of the actual physical wedge, but by the angle between an isodose curve and a line perpendicular to the central axis or at a specific depth
- There are a variety of definitions of where the wedge angle is found:
  - » At the 50 percent isodose curve
  - » At the 80 percent isodose curve
  - » At a depth of 10 cm
- Field sizes cannot be larger than the wedge itself
- Wedge transmission factor, or wedge factor, is added to the calculation of monitor units when a wedge is used
  - » It is measured on the central axis and ranges from 0.3 to 0.8
- Wedges "harden" the beam, meaning the low-energy photons are absorbed by the wedge, so a lower amount of photons are available for dose
  - » More MU is needed to compensate for the decrease of intensity, or the amount of photons
- Wedges reduce the dose rate

13. Off-Axis Calculation
   - Calculates the dose rate at a point in the field away from the central axis
   - The off-axis ratio (OAR) is the ratio of the dose rate at a point off-axis to the dose rate at a point on the central axis at the same distance from the source
   - A change in dose rate is expected toward the field edge due to the penumbra region
   - OAR values can be found on a lookup table
   - OARs can be used when the central axis is blocked by MLCs, blocks, or jaws for half-beam blocks

14. Isodose Curves and Their Characteristics
   - Isodose curves are a demonstration of the dose distribution within a field in directions parallel and perpendicular to the direction of the radiation beam
   - Each curve shows the percentage of dose at a specified depth
   - The curves are typically shown in increments of 10 percent
   - Factors that can change the isodose distribution are beam energy, source-to-surface distance, source-to-diaphragm distance, field weighting, and field size
   - A higher-energy beam's isodose curves are more spread out than lower-energy beams because the higher-energy beams are more penetrating
   - Wedges and patient contours can change the shape of the isodose curves
   - Dose-volume histograms (DVH) show the doses that normal tissue and tumors will receive during the treatment
      » Evaluated in three dimensions

15. Factors for Beam Modifiers
   - When blocks are needed for treatment, a tray made of some kind of plastic is used
      » The tray attenuates some of the beam (usually less than 5 percent)
      » When a tray is used, the MU must be increased to compensate for the attenuation of the beam
      » The tray factor (TF), or tray transmission factor, is a ratio of a dose with the tray in place to the dose without the tray and is found by a physicist
      » The tray transmission factor will change with different beam energies
   - Bolus is placed on the patient's skin
      » Located between the radiation beam and the skin
      » It brings the dose closer to the skin's surface and decreases skin sparing
      » Bolus will attenuate some of the beam
      » Does not require a factor to be added into the calculation for MU

- Wedges and compensators are used to alter the isodose distribution based on the patient's skin contour
  - » The transmission factor shows how much of the beam is transmitted through the wedge or compensator
  - » The transmission factor will change with changing beam energies
  - » The transmission factor will be different for each compensator because compensators are made specifically for each individual patient
  - » These factors are used when calculating for monitor units
  - » MU will likely increase with wedges and compensators because some of the original beam will be lost due to attenuation

16. Inhomogeneity
  - The dose distribution can change with tissue inhomogeneity
  - Different tissues have different densities and absorb the beam differently
  - Tissue inhomogeneities may cause scatter that can affect dose to other organs nearby
  - Tissues have a correction factor based on tissue types and electron density
  - The correction factors are applied to dose calculations to adjust for the dose distribution in different tissues

17. Rotational Fields
  - The maximum dose in full arcs, which rotate 360 degrees, is located in the isocenter
  - The maximum dose in partial arcs, which rotate less than 360 degrees, is located at a point between the isocenter and the skin's surface
    - » To adjust this so that the dose maximum is changed to be in the isocenter, the "past pointing" technique should be used
    - » Past pointing means the planner should point the beam past the preferred location for the dose maximum
  - TAR and TMR are used for dose rate calculations for rotational fields

18. Machine Output
  - The output factor compares the dose rate in a known field size to the dose rate in a reference field size
  - The output factor for the reference field size of 10x10 cm is 1.0
    - » For fields larger than 10x10 cm, the output factor will be greater than 1.0 due to an increase in scatter
    - » For fields smaller than 10x10 cm, the output factor will be less than 1.0 due to a decrease in scatter
  - Takes into account the amount of collimator scatter
  - The reference dose rate is 1.0 cGy/MU for linear accelerators and typically does not change

Part 4: Oncology Treatments

A. Types of Available Tratments

1. Chemotherapy

- Chemotherapy is a systemic treatment, meaning it is used to treat the whole body
- Chemotherapy drugs are cytotoxic and can kill the primary tumor cell and other tumor cells that have spread through the body
- Can be given orally, intravenously, intra-arterially, intraperitoneally, intrathecally, or topically
  - » Intrathecal administration must be done by a doctor
  - » The way the chemotherapy is given depends on the type of chemotherapy that is prescribed
- Doxorubicin (Adriamycin) can cause cardiac toxicity
- Bleomycin can cause pulmonary toxicity
- Doxorubicin is a radiosensitizer and increases the effect of radiation
- Amifostine is a radioprotector and decreases the effect of radiation on healthy cells

- **Alkylating agents**
  - » Chemically similar to the structure of mustard gas
  - » Does not depend on a specific cell cycle to be effective
  - » Hinders the actions of nucleic acids
  - » Side effects: bone marrow depression, amenorrhea (women), azoospermia (men), carcinogenesis
  - » If an alkylating agent comes in contact with skin, it can cause a burn
  - » Examples: carboplatin, cisplatin, nitrogen mustard, cyclophosphamide, chlorambucil
- **Antimetabolites**
  - » Work by disturbing the formation of new nucleic acids
  - » Effective in specific cell cycles
  - » Most effective with rapidly dividing cells
  - » Side effects: GI toxicity, acute bone marrow suppression
  - » Examples: methotrexate, 5-FU
- **Antitumor antibiotics**
  - » Originate from microbial fermentation
  - » Hinders the transcription of DNA and RNA
  - » Does not depend on a specific cell cycle, but is most effective in the S and G2 phases
  - » Side effects: cardiac toxicity, skin ulceration, pulmonary toxicity, bone marrow suppression, increased effects of radiation therapy
  - » Examples: doxorubicin (Adriamycin), bleomycin, mitomycin C, actinomycin D
- **Hormonal agents**
  - » Remove or replace naturally occurring hormones
  - » Commonly used to treat breast cancer
  - » Side effects: hot flashes, depression, loss of libido, increased risk of endometrial cancer
  - » Examples: tamoxifen, corticosteroids (dexamethasone, hydrocortisone, prednisone), leuprolide

- **Nitrosoureas**
  - » Similar to alkylating agents because they hinder the synthesis of DNA
  - » Does not depend on a specific cell cycle to be effective
  - » Lipid soluble
  - » Has the ability to cross the blood-brain barrier
  - » Side effects: delayed myelosuppression, GI toxicity, delayed nephrotoxicity
  - » Examples: carmustine, lomustine, streptozocin
- **Vinca alkaloids**
  - » Originate from the periwinkle plant
  - » Terminate cell replication in metaphase
  - » Side effects: neurotoxicity, skin ulceration, myelosuppression
  - » Examples: vincristine, vinblastine, etoposide

Common chemotherapy used for specific cancers as stated by Kole:

Anal cancer	5-FU, Mitomycin, Capecitabine
Bladder cancer	5-FU, Cisplatin, Gemcitabine
Esophageal cancer	5-FU, Mitomycin, Cisplatin, Carboplatin, Taxol
Head and neck cancers	5-FU, Cisplatin, Taxol, Carboplatin
Hodgkin's	ABVD (Adriamycin, Bleomycin, Vinblastine, Dacarbazine), MOPP (Nitrogen Mustard, Oncovin, Prednisone, Procarbazine), and BEACOPP (Bleomycin, Etoposide, Doxorubicine, Cyclophosphamide, Vincristine, Prednisone, Procarbazine)
Pancreatic cancers	5-FU, Oxaliplatin, Gemcitabine
Rectal cancer	5-FU, Oxaliplatin, Leucovorin
Non-small cell lung cancer	Cisplatin, Carboplatin, Etoposide, Taxol, Pemetrexed
Brain cancer	Temozolomide
Breast cancer	Taxel, Carboplatin, CMF (Cyclophosphamide, Methotrexate, 5-FU)

2. <u>Surgery</u>
- Surgery is used to treat tumors locally
- Used to diagnose, stage, and treat tumors, and for palliative care
- Surgical biopsies diagnosis and stage tumors
  - » Some methods for biopsy are fine-needle aspiration, core needle, endoscopic, incisional, and excisional
- The outcome of surgery depends on the patient's medical condition and the size, extent, and location of the tumor
  - » Surgeries of smaller tumors have better outcomes
- Surgery is difficult for nasopharyngeal tumors due to their inaccessible location
  - » This area is in close proximity to the base of brain and cranial nerves
- Risks of having surgery are the harmful reactions to anesthesia, infection, and partial or complete loss of organ function

3. Radiation Therapy

a. External Beam

- A local treatment for tumors
- Radiation treatments can preserve the function of organs and lead to better cosmetic outcomes as compared with surgery
- Not all organs and areas can benefit from radiation therapy
  - » Restricted to areas where the dose needed to eradicate the tumor can be delivered without harming normal tissues
- Use x-rays, electrons, protons, or gamma rays
  - » X-rays are manmade (electrons hit a target)
  - » Gamma rays are created through radioactive decay

b. Brachytherapy

- "Short-distance therapy"
- Radioactive source is positioned next to the tumor or within the tumor
- Sustains the surrounding healthy tissue
- Examples of radioactive materials are cesium-137, iridium-192, palladium-103, or iodine-125
- Activity formula: $A = A_o \, e(-0.693/t_{1/2}) \times (t)$
  - » A = activity
  - » A_o = initial activity
  - » $t_{1/2}$ = half life
  - » t = time
- Decay constant $\lambda = 0.693/t_{1/2}$
- Mean life = $1.44 \times (t_{1/2})$
- **Interstitial implants:** the source is positioned within the tumor
  - » Permanent or temporary
  - » Can be used for prostate, head and neck, or breast cancers
- **Intracavitary implants:** the source is positioned within a body cavity
  - » Can be used for cervical or endometrial cancers
  - » The applicator may be positioned surgically
  - » Low-dose implants are placed within patients for long periods of time, and the patient must stay within the hospital as an inpatient
  - » High-dose implants are placed within patients for short periods of time in multiple fractions and the patient can leave the hospital between fractions
- **Intraluminal implants:** the source is placed within a body tube like the esophagus or bronchus
  - » Removed from the patient when the prescribed dose has been delivered
- **Intravascular implants:** the source is placed within a vessel and it avoids the narrowing of blood vessels after angioplasty

4. Multimodality

- Concomitant or concurrent treatment is when two different kinds of treatments occur at the same time
- Sequential treatment is when one treatment option follows another treatment (one after the other)
- Adjuvant treatment is a treatment given in addition to the primary treatment

5. Immunotherapy

- A cancer treatment that uses the body's defense system to fight cancerous tumors
- Immunotherapy activates the body's own immune system to work harder and fight the cancer cells
- Immunotherapy can also be the addition of man-made substances that were created in a laboratory
- This treatment can slow the growth of the tumor, reduce the spread of the cancer, and help the immune system fight against the cancer
- Some types of immunotherapy can train the body's immune system to attack only cancerous cells
- This does not work for every type of cancer
- Still a newer treatment and under a lot of research

B. Treatment Verification

1. Patient Position

- The patient's position should be reproducible for each treatment
- The patient should be positioned as straight and level as possible
  » This is achieved through triangulation
  » The patient is typically given two or three tattoos
  » The tattoos will be aligned using the lasers on the wall and ceiling to position the patient in the same exact way they were lying for their simulation
- There may be various shifts to move the table and patient to specific coordinates, which brings the patient into treatment position
  » The table is moved in the x, y, and z directions to help line up the isocenter
- The patient must be in a comfortable position and unlikely to move during treatment
- Explanation of the patient's position should be clearly located in the chart so it can be reproduced daily
  » Immobilization devices, positioning aids, external landmarks, indexing locations, and tattoos should be explained
  » Other ways to describe positioning (like supine, prone, arm arrangement and location of positioning devices) should be included
  » Known measurements like table top or anatomical measurements should be noted as well
- The patient needs to take off any devices that would be in the treatment field
  » Examples: dentures, hearing aids
- If prescribed, internal shielding is placed before the patient is positioned for treatment

2. Isocenter
  - The isocenter is located where the vertical and horizontal lasers meet
  - The isocenter is a point that the gantry, couch, and collimator rotate around

3. Machine Setup
  - The gantry and collimator are positioned according to the parameters created during the treatment planning
    » They are positioned to get the best isodose distribution to the tumor while sparing critical structures as much as possible
  - Treatment field sizes depend on the size of the tumor, nodal involvement, and critical structures
  - The field size is defined at the isocenter
  - The energy is determined during treatment planning
    » Measurements must be taken during the simulation (or after, using the CT simulation images) to determine depth of the tumor and patient separation
    » The depth of the tumor will help determine which energy to use to ensure enough coverage of dose to the tumor

4. Prescription
  - Radiation treatments are prescribed by a radiation oncologist
  - A patient's prescription must be written and signed before the treatment starts
  - The prescription will include the anatomic site, total dose, fractionation dose, fractionation schedule, beam energy, respiratory gating (if necessary), and devices such as bolus
  - The prescription may change during the patient's course of radiation
  - It is important for the radiation therapist to be aware of these changes before they treat the patient

5. Modality
  a. 2-D
  - Conventional treatment planning
  - Uses a conventional simulator with x-ray equipment
  - Provides a radiographic image with an outline of the tumor and a small margin
  - Dose distributions are limited to single fields or a few fields

  b. 3-D
  - Three-dimensional treatment plan
  - Uses a CT simulator
  - Anatomy and critical structures are more accurately defined
  - More optimized dose distributions compared with 2-D treatment plans
  - Dose volume histograms (DVH) and digitally reconstructed radiographs (DRRs) are created
    » More accurate patient positioning

c. 4-D

- Four-dimensional treatment plan
- Incorporates respiratory motion into 3-D treatment planning
- Demonstrates the motion of the tumor during the breathing cycle
- An ITV (internal treatment volume) may be made to include the full length the target will travel in the breathing cycles
- Respiratory gating can also be used
  - » The radiation beam is on when the tumor is within a specific treatment position; the beam is turned off when the tumor moves out of the treatment position
  - » Tumor location can be known through various monitors

d. IMRT

- Intensity-Modulated Radiation Therapy
- Advanced version of 3-D treatment planning
- Creates a nonuniform radiation beam in order to optimize the dose to the tumor while minimizing the dose to organs at risk near the tumor
- Uses complex treatment planning (forward or inverse)
  - » **Inverse planning:** maximum dose to the tumor and maximum dose to organs at risk are defined
    - This information helps the computer create MLC patterns and dose distributions
    - This is the treatment planning used for IMRT
  - » **Forward planning:** beam parameters and modifiers are added to the treatment plan first and then the dose distribution is reviewed
    - The parameters can be changed until the plan is optimal
    - Trial-and-error method (not used for IMRT)

e. Arc/Rotational Therapy

- Rotational fields are also known as arc therapy, where the radiation is delivered while the gantry is moving in an arc from one set point to another
- For arcs less than 360 degrees, the treatment planning method is called past pointing
  - » The treatment plans for the beam to treat to a depth farther than the center of the tumor
- For arcs that are 360 degrees, the beam is set to treat at the exact depth of the center of the tumor
- Arc speed is calculated as MU/degree
- Before treating with an arc, the therapist should do a dry run of the gantry rotation to ensure there will be no collisions between the gantry and the patient or table

f. Stereotactic Radiosurgery

- Stereotactic radiosurgery is a single-fraction, high-dose radiation therapy
  - » Typically treats tumors in the cranium
- A stereotactic head frame is attached to the patient's skull for the day
  - » This creates a landmark for accurate localization
- Radiosurgery is planned when CT and MRI studies are fused or registered
- Accurate to about 0.5 to 1.0 mm

6. Imaging Procedures

   a. kV Imaging
   - kV imaging uses an onboard kV imager to image the patient prior to treatment when the patient is in their treatment position
   - kV images are 2-D
   - When kV images are at taken every treatment, it is considered an IGRT treatment (image guided radiation therapy)
     » An orthogonal pair is taken (two images taken at perpendicular angles from each other)
       - Example: AP & lateral
       - The gantry moves around the patient to obtain images at each angle
   - kV images are more detailed and have better contrast than MV images
   - kV images are compared against DRRs
     » Digitally reconstructed radiographs (DRRs) are created from data obtained during the CT scan and show radiographic landmarks like bony anatomy
     » Shifts can be made from the images before each treatment

   b. Cone Beam CT (CBCT)
   - CBCT images are 3-D or volumetric images
   - Multiple images are taken at different gantry angles, which are then reconstructed to create a 3-D image
   - After reconstruction, these images can be viewed in three planes
     » Axial, sagittal, and coronal
   - The 3-D images from the CBCT can be compared with the original 3-D images from the time of the CT simulation
     » This is known as registration

   c. MV Imaging
   - MV imaging takes portal images
   - The portal is also known as the treatment field, or the area exposed to radiation
   - Portal imaging is taken in the beam's-eye view (BEV), or from the angle and setting the patient will be treated with
   - Verifies the patient's position and the collimation or aperture settings
   - Ensures an accurate treatment
   - Portal images are compared with DRRs for verification
   - Portal imaging is done before treatments start to verify the treatment plan and then at certain increments throughout treatment as specified on the prescription
     » Most common is weekly, or once every five fractions
   - Port films are created from MV photons, and images are less clear due to the high rate of Compton scatter
     » Limited contrast
     » Identifying radiographic landmarks is more difficult with MV images compared with kV images

C. Treatment Setup

1. <u>Devices Used During Patient Setup</u>

   a. *Indexing*
   - Positioning devices are locked into a specific location on the treatment table
   - There are notches at specific increments on the treatment table that allow an "index bar" to be locked in
     » Wing boards, breast boards, head and neck boards, u-frame head holders, etc. can lock into the index bar
   - Makes treatment setup and patient positioning more accurate and reproducible each day

   b. *Positioning Aids*
   - Help to position the patient for treatment
   - They do not constrain the patient's movement
   - Can be reused for multiple patients
   - Examples: head holders, sponge pillows, foam cushions, neck rolls

   c. *Lasers*
   - Lasers are mounted on the walls and ceiling to help level and line up the patient to the treatment position
   - The side lasers are located on the walls on each side of the gantry
     » Lasers are a fan beam in vertical and horizontal planes
     » They make sure the patient is leveled correctly
   - The sagittal laser is located on the wall opposite the gantry
     » Laser is a fan beam in the vertical plane
     » Helps align the patient to the axis of the table
   - The ceiling laser is located on the ceiling above the gantry
     » Aims vertically down toward the isocenter
   - Lasers are either solid-state diode lasers or helium-neon gas lasers
   - Lasers are checked daily and have a tolerance of 2 mm

2. <u>Machine Capabilities</u>

   a. *SSD Versus SAD*
   - Linear accelerators can treat patients with SSD or SAD treatments
   - For SSD treatments, the patient's skin is placed at a fixed distance from the source
     » The patient must be moved in between treatment fields to maintain the fixed distance
   - For SAD treatments, the patient is positioned so that the isocenter is located within the patient's body
     » The SSD will read a number lower than 100 cm
       - Depends on the depth of the tumor or the patient's separation
     » The patient does not need to be moved between treatment fields

b. Collimator and Electron Cone Parameters

- The secondary collimators are moveable and can create asymmetric rectangular fields
- Field sizes range from 0x0 cm to 40x40 cm
  - » Measured at the isocenter
- Collimators are typically made of tungsten
- Less than 0.5 percent of the beam is allowed to be transmitted through the collimator jaws
- Collimator rotates around the central axis and isocenter
- Collimator and MLCs delineate the treatment field
- For electron therapy, cones are used because electrons scatter easily in air
- Cones collimate the electrons close to the skin's surface
- An electron cutout must be made to fit within the cone to further collimate the beam
  - » Cutouts can be customized for the patient or predetermined shapes like circles
- Electron cones come in multiple field sizes: 6x6 cm, 10x10 cm, 15x15 cm (14x14 cm for Elekta), 20x20 cm and 25x25 cm

c. Optical or Mechanical Distance Indicator

- Optical distance indicator (ODI) is also known as the "range finder"
- Displays a light with a scale in centimeters on the patient's surface to specify the SSD
- Located on or near the collimator
- The ODI has a ± 2 mm tolerance and is checked daily before treatments
- The mechanical distance indicator is a physical ruler
- When the ODI is not working, the mechanical indicator can be used in its place to check the SSD
- More commonly, the mechanical distance indicator is used for QA checks
  - » It checks the ODI, gantry angle, and collimator angle

d. Gantry Angle

- The gantry can rotate 360 degrees around the isocenter
- The radiation beam can be delivered from just about every angle
- The term "en face" is used when the gantry is parallel to the patient's skin or contour
  - » The central axis is perpendicular to the patient
  - » Used for electron beams and clinical setups
- The gantry, collimator, and couch rotate around the isocenter

e. Collimator Angle

- The collimator can rotate 360 degrees around the isocenter
- Collimator angles are typically reversed for parallel opposed fields
  - » Example: the collimator is 30 degrees for the left lateral brain field and 330 degrees for the right lateral brain field

f. Field Light
- A field light is projected from the collimator to represent the radiation field
- The divergence and shape of the field light are the same as the radiation field
- A QA test is done monthly to check the field light accuracy to the radiation field
- There is a 2 mm tolerance
- The QA test is checked with a "ready pack" film

g. Treatment Couch
- The treatment couch is also called the "patient support assembly" (PSA) or "pedestal"
- The couch has the ability to move vertically (up and down), laterally (side to side), and longitudinally (in and out)
- The couch can also rotate from the vertical axis
  - » Also referred to as "couch kicks"
- The PSA is made out of carbon fiber
- It should be lightweight, flat, and firm for a reproducible setup
- Older couches are made with a mesh with clear plastic over it at the top, which decreases attenuation of the beam and allows for more radiation to travel through the couch
- Newer couches allow the table to adjust for roll, pitch, and yaw (6 degrees of freedom)

h. Console Controls
- The radiation therapist controls the radiation delivery from the treatment console
- It is located outside of the treatment room behind appropriate shielding
- The console shows the treatment parameters for each patient according to the record and verify system and the status of the treatment machine
- The console will alert the therapist of any interlocks, which are safety precautions and will stop the beam from turning on
  - » Example: wrong accessories (like wedges, compensators, and electron cones), collisions, open door, etc.
- The gantry and collimator can be moved from the treatment console if the treatment door is closed
- The imagers can be moved from the treatment console
- Dose rate, MU, field sizes, gantry angle, collimator angle, couch angle, and accessories are examples of what is shown on the treatment console

i. Pendant Controls
- The pendant is located within the treatment room and is attached to the treatment couch
- The pendant allows the radiation therapist to control the table and gantry motions
  - » Vertical, lateral, longitudinal, and couch kick/rotation movements of the couch
  - » The gantry and collimator can also be rotated using the pendant
- Using the pendant, the therapist has the ability to open or close field sizes temporarily
  - » This will not change the field size for the patient's treatment, but they can open up field sizes to help visualize SSDs or anything else they may need
- Imagers can also be moved using the pendants in the room

» There are options to move the MV images, KV imagers, or both
- The room lights, field lights, ODI and lasers can be turned on and off using the pendant
- Newer machines have pendants equipped with a flashlight to help visualize patient marks and tattoos better for treatment setup
- The pendant will only function if the user is holding down the two side bars known as the "dead man switch"
    » There is one bar on each side of the pendant
    » If they are not pressed down or engaged, the motions will not enable
    » This is an extra safety precaution

D. Treatment Machine Accessories

1. Beam Modifiers

    a. Compensating Filters
    - Compensators are meant to create a homogeneous isodose distribution within the patient
    - Placed in between the source of radiation and the patient to modify the radiation beam and to compensate for the patient's skin contour
    - Made with a high-density material, such as Cerrobend or "poly lead"
    - Custom-made for each individual patient
    - Most useful when treating areas of the body with a lot of skin sloping, such as the head and neck, AP lung, and breast
    - Two types of compensators: missing tissue compensators and dose compensators
        » A **missing tissue compensator** makes up for a sloping skin surface and creates a more homogeneous dose distribution
        » A **dose compensator** makes up for missing tissue and inhomogeneities in the patient's anatomy
    - In order to create a compensator for the patient, there must be a skin topography, which is created with data from the CT scan
    - The thickness of the compensator is determined by factors like beam divergence, the compensator material's linear attenuation coefficient, and scatter
    - Compensators for photon therapy must be placed at least 20 cm from the patient's skin to reduce scatter to the skin's surface and therefore maintain skin sparing
    - Compensators for electron therapy are placed directly on the patient
    - When calculating the dose rate and using a compensator, a transmission factor must be included
    - Today, compensators have typically been replaced by IMRT (intensity modulated radiation therapy)

    b. Treatment Shields
    - **Internal shields:** used during electron therapy to shield critical structures that are located directly behind the tumor being treated
        » Used when treating thin, superficial tumors (located in areas such as eyelids, nostrils, earlobes, and lips) that have organs at risk directly behind them (such as oral mucosa, nasal membranes, optic lens, lacrimal glands, and gingiva)
        » Lead shields alone will cause backscatter when the beam interacts with it, which

causes the dose to escalate

» Therefore, internal shields must be covered with a material of low Z number to absorb the scatter

- A common combination used is lead covered by wax
- Other common materials used are aluminum and plastic
- Eye shields are made of tungsten with an aluminum cap

- **Transmission filters:** limit a certain percentage of the beam to pass through at a certain location within the treatment field

» Helpful with certain organs that are more radiosensitive within the field

» Allows the patient to be more tolerant of the treatment

c. Blocks

- **Hand blocks:** premade shields created with a high-density material
  » Not customized for each patient
  » Prefabricated shapes (example: kidney shape)
  » Placed on or bolted onto a tray that is placed in the accessory holder
  » Typically used in emergency situations when cast blocks cannot be made in time
  » Positioned on a tray using the light field and shadows on the patient
  » Hand blocks are non-divergent, so the angle of the sides of the block do not match the angle of the beam, which creates penumbra

- **Cast blocks:** shields that are individualized for each patient
  » Can be created into almost any shape
  » Secured onto the block tray in a specific position
  » When cast blocks are made for the patient, they are cut to match the angle of the divergence of the radiation beam in order to reduce penumbra
  » Made of Cerrobend, or "Lipowitz's metal"
    - Cerrobend is made up of 50 percent bismuth, 26.7 percent lead, 13.3 percent tin, and 10 percent cadmium
    - Cerrobend has a lower melting point than lead and melts at 74°C (165°F)

- Transmission of the radiation beam through the cast block is less than 5 percent
- The thickness of Cerrobend blocks ranges from 6 to 8 cm
  » Most common thickness is 7.5 cm

- **Positive** blocks are blocks that shield more of the central part of the radiation field, leaving the periphery open
  » Example: lung blocks

- **Negative blocks** are blocks that shield the periphery of the radiation field and the central portion is open
  » Example: electron cutouts

- Blocks used with photon beams should be placed at a minimum of 20 cm from the surface of the patient
  » This will reduce scatter and any unwanted extra skin dose

d. Multileaf Collimators

- Metal leaves that collimate and shape the treatment field
- 52 to 160 motorized tungsten leaves located in the treatment head of the linear accelerator
- Each leaf can move independently to create a wide variety of treatment field shapes
  » Controlled by a computer
- Field shapes are customized for each patient and treatment field
- Reduces the need for cast blocks
  » Blocks are sometimes still needed for "island blocks" for areas like the kidney that are in the middle of the treatment field
- Leaf width varies from 0.4 to 2.0 cm
  » The narrower the width of the leaf, the more conformal the shape of the beam can be
- Transmission through the MLC is less than 2 percent
- IMRT is possible with the use of MLCs
- In IMRT, there are two methods:
  » **Step and shoot:** the beam is delivered with MLCs in one stationary position, turned off as the MLCs reposition to the next segment, and then turned back on
  » **Dynamic:** the beam remains on as the MLCs and gantry move throughout the treatment
    - Also known as a "sliding window"

e. Bolus

- Bolus is used to eliminate skin-sparing effects in photon therapy, compensate for irregular surface contours, and eliminate air gaps in treatment fields
- Made of materials similar to tissue or water
- Bolus is placed over the treatment area to absorb some of the build up dose so the d_{max} is more superficial
- Most commonly used when treating tumors that are superficial, tumors in the skin, scars, and superficial lymph nodes
- Bolus should be flexible and able to conform to the patient's contour
  » There should be no air gaps between the bolus and patient
- Examples of bolus material are superflab, wet gauze, wet towels, paraffin wax, Vaseline gauze, etc.
- Bolus is available in varying thicknesses
- The use of bolus will be prescribed by the Radiation Oncologist

f. Wedges

- Wedges help reduce hot spots in treatment plans with multiple fields with hinge angles less than 180
- Wedges are used for tissue compensation of sloping surfaces such as breasts
- Standard wedges can be slid into the collimator of the gantry externally
  » Made out of steel or lead
- Dynamic wedges are created by moving one jaw (usually the Y-jaw) as the beam is delivered

- The thick end of a wedge is called the "heel"; it absorbs or attenuates more of the beam than the "toe," or the thin end of the wedge
    » Wedges are oriented "heel to heel" or "toe to toe"
    » The heel end of the wedge brings the isodose curves up higher to the surface within the patient
- Common wedges: 15, 30, 45, and 60 degrees

2. Immobilization
    a. Custom Immobilization Devices
    - Custom immobilization devices can be used only for the one specific patient they were made for
    - Examples of custom immobilization devices are Alpha Cradles, Vac-Lok, and Aquaplast
    - **Alpha Cradle:** immobilization cast made of a foaming agent like polyurethane and a Styrofoam base
        » It is created by mixing liquid chemicals and pouring them into a plastic bag; the patient then lies on the bag in the treatment position and the chemicals expand and foam up to conform to the patient's body
        » The chemicals take about ten minutes to harden
        » Can be used to immobilize many body parts, but most frequently used for breast, thorax, and lower extremity treatments
        » Custom made for each patient and cannot be reused
    - **Vac-Lok:** immobilization device that uses a vacuum and small beads of Styrofoam within a thick plastic bag
        » The bag is positioned underneath the patient in the treatment position
        » The small beads within the plastic bag conform to the patient's body and air is vacuumed out, enabling the Vac-Lok to hold the patient's shape
        » Can be reused after the patient is done and the Vac-Lok is cleaned
    - **Aquaplast:** thermoplastic mold
        » When warmed in hot water, the thermoplastic becomes flexible and can be molded around the patient's contour
            - Material becomes flexible and clear at temperatures of 70°C to 80°C (160°F-180°F)
            - After it has been removed from the water for 10 minutes, the material will cool and looks opaque
        » Available in solid form or mesh form and in different thicknesses
        » Commonly used to immobilize patients for head and neck or brain treatments
        » The thermoplastic mold must be connected to a head frame or baseplate that is attached to the treatment table so it does not move

b. Basic Immobilization Devices
- Standard or basic immobilization devices can be used for multiple patients
- Must be cleaned before each patient's use
- Head holders, sponge pillows, foam cushions, and neck rolls are used to help with immobilization and are not custom to the patient; can be used for multiple patients
- A prone breast board is an elevated board with a cushion over it and a window cut out for the breast to fall through for treatment
  » This allows the breast that is to be treated to hang lower than the rest of the patient's body
  » Used for pendulous and large breasts
  » This board can be used for many different patients
- A belly board is a cushion or mattress with a window cut out in the middle so that when the patient lies prone, the abdomen can hang down
  » Allows the intestines to hang low and away from the lateral fields, which will lower the dose delivered to the intestines
  » Used to treat pelvic tumors such as the rectum
- Wing boards and breast boards are used to place the patient in the supine position with the arms above the heads
  » Used for multiple patients
  » Can place custom immobilization devices over this, such as a Vac-Lok or Alpha Cradle

E. Treatment Application
1. Patient Monitoring Systems
   a. Visual
   - Therapist does not directly see the patient, but can visualize them through TV monitors
   - Used for megavoltage units
   - TV monitors are constantly on so that a visual connection occurs at all times
   - Typically, at least two cameras are on for each treatment
     » One camera shows a long view of the patient and shows the whole body
     » The other camera is closer to show subtler movements
   - If there is no visualization and the TV monitors are malfunctioning, treatment cannot occur

   b. Two-Way Audio Communication
   - While the patient is in the treatment room and the therapists are at the treatment console, audio contact must be possible at all times
   - There is a two-way communication system between the treatment room and the treatment console
   - The therapists constantly hear inside the treatment room while at the console
   - However, the therapists must press a button or hit a switch to speak into the treatment room when necessary
     » The patient cannot constantly hear the therapists at the treatment console
     » The patient can hear the therapist only when the button is pressed

c. Backup Software
- Malfunctions can happen during treatments from mechanical or electronic trouble
- Devices must be repaired prior to treating patients
- Backup counters record the amount of monitor units that were delivered before a power failure occurred
  » Backup counters have an independent power supply, such as a battery, so when there is a power failure to the department the counter still functions
- The amount of monitor units must be recorded when a malfunction occurs so that the patient can finish their treatment appropriately when the machine works properly

2. Record and Verify Systems
- The R&V system is software that allows communication between the treatment planning system and the linear accelerator control system
- Displays the parameters of the machine setup from the treatment plan and compares it with what the machine is set to at that time
  » Machine will not turn on if parameters do not match and are out of a known tolerance
- Examples of the parameters that are displayed are MU, gantry angle, collimator angle, field size, table position, and beam modifiers
- The R&V system also records each treatment for each patient
- If images are taken, the R&V system will record the couch parameters and any shifts made during the imaging process

3. Image Matching/Registration
- There are many methods to obtain images in radiation therapy
- The appropriate method to be used is directed by the physician's prescription
- Image registration is the matching of the images taken on the day of treatment to the DRR or the CT
  » Digitally reconstructed radiographs (DRRs) are created from data obtained during the CT scan and show radiographic landmarks like bony anatomy
  » The original CT simulation images are used to compare and register the patient's CBCT
- Images are compared "side by side" with the DRR or they can be "blended" with one image on top of the other
- **Online image review** means the images are reviewed before treatment
  » Typically, the therapist reviews the images before treatment so that the necessary adjustments can be made to the setup to ensure maximum accuracy
- **Offline image review** means the images are reviewed after treatment
  » Typically, the doctor checks the images offline
  » Offline images must be approved before the next treatment takes places
- This process verifies the patient position and ensures an accurate treatment

- **Portal imaging:** taken in the beam's-eye view (BEV)
  - » The portal is also known as the treatment field, or the area exposed to radiation
  - » Verifies the collimation or aperture settings
  - » Portal images are compared with DRRs for verification
  - » Portal imaging is done before treatments start to verify the treatment plan and then at certain increments throughout the treatment as specified on the prescription
  - » Most common is weekly, or once every five fractions
  - » Port films are created from MV photons and images are less clear due to the high rate of Compton scatter
- **Electronic portal imaging devices (EPIDs):** newer technology that uses flat-panel x-ray detectors
  - » EPIDs are ready to be reviewed immediately and do not have to be processed like films
  - » Images are evaluated and adjustments can be made quicker
  - » The image quality can be improved by adjusting window and level
- **Image guided radiation therapy (IGRT):** images the patient's soft tissue or tissue markers before treatment to verify an accurate treatment
  - » Onboard kV imagers, CBCT, CT on rails, MV CT, ultrasound, etc.
  - » Compares images with DRRs or CT axial slices (known as registering)
    - • Can make small table adjustments to better align the patient
  - » kV images have better quality and less scatter than MV images

4. Treatment Port Verification
  - • The way to verify the site to be treated is through imaging
  - • After the patient has been triangulated, they must be imaged before the treatment begins
  - • All portals must be imaged using a double exposure
    - » The first exposure shows the treatment field and MLCs
    - » The second exposure is taken after the collimator jaws are opened more so that more anatomy can be seen for comparison/registration
  - • Depending on the angles of the port fields, an additional orthogonal pair may be needed to verify the isocenter
    - » The anterior field will verify the position in the superior to inferior direction as well as the lateral directions
    - » The lateral field will verify the position in the anterior to posterior as well as superior to inferior directions
      - • Verifies that you are treating at the correct depth

5. Verification of Treatment Dose
- The dose can be verified with diodes because they can provide a real-time reading
  - » Diodes are used for patient dosimetry
  - » Placed on the surface of the patient in the treatment field
  - » Diodes are attached to an electrometer to display dose
- Other ways to verify dose are TLDs (thermoluminescent dosimeters) and MOSFETs (metal-oxide semiconductor field-effect transistors)
- Film can also verify dose
  - » Optical density (blackness of the film) correlates with dose
  - » Permanent record of dose

6. Treatment Machine Malfunctions
  a. Types
  - Some types of equipment hazards are electrical, radiation, software, and mechanical
  - Examples: radiation overdose, dose to the wrong area due to equipment malfunctions, incorrect energy, lack of beam symmetry or flatness, etc.

  b. How To Adjust When There Is A Malfunction
  - Some interlocks do not require immediate attention
    - » In some cases the therapist may be able to clear a fault temporarily and continue treating
      - Example: a fault in the couch motion during setup
    - » If the same fault occurs at a rate such as one or more per treatment, the treatments should be stopped until a service engineer can repair the machine
    - » These faults must be reported to the physicist and the service engineer
  - The therapist may be able to clear faults by resetting the machine
  - If this does not work, the machine cannot operate and must be fixed by the physicist or service engineer
    - » The physicist or service engineer then has to try to duplicate the fault and figure out why it occurred and how to fix it
    - » Very rarely, the physicist may need to recalibrate the machine

  c. Documentating Malfunctions
  - Equipment malfunctions need to be reported to the radiation oncologist and radiation physicist and should also be documented
  - The radiation physicist is primarily responsible for documenting
  - If the malfunction leads to a misadministration of the radiation, it must be reported by the guidelines of the state or the guidelines of the Nuclear Regulatory Commission (NRC)
  - If the equipment malfunction causes a severe injury or death, it must be reported to the U.S. Food and Drug Administration per the Medical Device Reporting Act

Helpful Math Formulas

1. MU SSD = $\dfrac{\text{Dose}}{\text{Everything Else x (PDD)}}$

"Everything Else" means any other important output factors given in the question Examples: wedge factor, tray factor, scatter factor, etc.

2. MU SAD = $\dfrac{\text{Dose}}{\text{Everything Else x (TMR)}}$

3. MU Electrons = $\dfrac{\text{Dose}}{\text{Everything Else x (Normalization Factor)}}$

4. MU Extended Distance = $\dfrac{\text{Dose x (Inverse Square Factor)}}{\text{(Cone Factor) x (Normalization Factor)}}$

5. Magnification Factor = $\dfrac{\text{Source to Film Distance}}{\text{Source to Object Distance}} = \dfrac{\text{Size on Film}}{\text{Actual Size}}$

6. Maynord "F" Factor = $\left(\dfrac{SSD_2 + d_{max}}{SSD_1 + d_{max}} \text{ x } \dfrac{SSD_1 + \text{depth}}{SSD_2 + \text{depth}} \right)^2$ x old PDD to get new PDD

7. Equivalent Square = $\dfrac{2\,(a \text{ x } b)}{a + b} = \dfrac{4 \text{ x area}}{\text{Perimeter}}$

   a = length of one side of a rectangle
   b = length of other side of a rectangle (perpendicular to "a")

8. Blocked Equivalent Square = $\sqrt{\text{(Area of Open Field) - (Area of Blocked Field)}}$

   = Open Equivalent Square x $\sqrt{1 - \text{(\% of Blocked Area)}}$

9. Dose at D_{max} or "Applied Dose" = $\dfrac{\text{Total Dose}}{\text{PDD}}$

10. Dose at underlying structure (not D_{max}) = Applied dose x PDD at specified organ

11. Wedge Angle = $90 - \dfrac{\text{Hinge Angle}}{2}$

125

12. Hinge Angle = 180 - (Wedge Angle x 2)

13. Gap Calculation = $\dfrac{\text{Depth}}{2}\left(\dfrac{L_1}{SSD_1} + \dfrac{L_2}{SSD_2}\right)$

$\qquad\qquad = \dfrac{\text{Depth}}{2}\left(\dfrac{L_1}{SSD_1}\right) + \left(\dfrac{L_2}{SSD_2}\right)$

      L = field length

14. Collimator Rotation for CranioSpinal Irraditation = Arctan $\emptyset$ $\dfrac{1}{2}\left(\dfrac{L_1}{SSD_1}\right)$

      L_1 = length of spinal field

15. Couch Rotation for CranioSpinal Irraditation = Arctan $\emptyset$ $\dfrac{1}{2}\left(\dfrac{L_2}{SAD}\right)$

      L_2 = length of lateral crianial field

16. Inverse Square Law $\quad \dfrac{I_1}{I_2} = \left(\dfrac{D_2}{D_1}\right)^2$

17. Inverse Square Factor = $\left(\dfrac{SSD_1}{SSD_2}\right)^2$

18. Electrons: 80% isodose line = $\dfrac{\text{MeV}}{3}$

                    90% isodose line = $\dfrac{\text{MeV}}{4}$

                    Useful range = $\dfrac{\text{MeV}}{2}$

                    Cutout thickness (in mm) = $\dfrac{\text{MeV}}{2} + 1$

19. Arc Rotation = $\dfrac{\text{MU}}{\text{MU/degree}}$

20. To find "cGy/degree" = $\dfrac{\text{cGy}}{\text{Total degrees of gantry rotation}}$

21. Therapeutic Ratio = $\dfrac{\text{Normal Tissue Tolerance Dose}}{\text{Tumor Lethal Dose}}$

22. Tissue Weighting = MU x $\dfrac{\text{Weight of field}}{\text{Sum of all weights}}$

23. Mean Life = 1.44 x $T_{1/2}$

    T = time

24. Mean Energy = 1/3 x Peak Energy

25. Block Thickness $\dfrac{1}{2^n}$ = % of transmission desired

    n = number of HVLs

Practice Test 1

1. An immobilization device that is made of foaming agents is known as:
   a. Alpha cradles
   b. Vac-Lok
   c. Aquaplast
   d. Cerrobend

2. Comparing CBCT images to the CT simulation images and making adjustments is known as:
   a. Registration
   b. Representation
   c. Rendering
   d. Recording

3. If the radiation worker is expected to receive _____ of effective dose, they should be monitored.
   a. 10%
   b. 20%
   c. 30%
   d. 40%

4. Which type of leukemia does NOT use bone marrow transplants as a form of treatment?
   a. ALL
   b. AML
   c. CLL
   d. CML

5. Which of the following is NOT assessed during a complete blood count blood study?
   a. Plasma
   b. Hemoglobin
   c. Hematocrit
   d. Glucose

6. Which of the following is NOT a primary component of Cerrobend?
   a. Lead
   b. Tin
   c. Bismuth
   d. Cerium

7. Brachytherapy is use for:
   a. Short distance radiation therapy
   b. External beam radiation therapy
   c. Extended distance radiation therapy
   d. Stereotactic radiation therapy

8. A patient is receiving arc therapy for 27 treatments. The total dose is 54 Gy, with a daily dose of 200 cGy. The arc will deliver 250 MU. The gantry is moving 360 degrees. Calculate the arc speed.
   a. 0.56 MU/degree
   b. 0.69 MU/degree
   c. 1.44 MU/degree
   d. 1.80 MU degree

9. The legal doctrine that states the employer is liable for the employee's negligence is known as:
   a. Respondeat superior
   b. Res ipsa loquitur
   c. Tort
   d. Res ipsa superior

10. If a lymphoma spreads in a random pattern, it is most likely:
    a. Hodgkin's
    b. Non-Hodgkin's
    c. Chronic
    d. Acute

11. What is the tolerance dose to 1/3 of the kidney according to Emami et al.?
    a. 2300 cGy
    b. 3000 cGy
    c. 4500 cGy
    d. 5000 cGy

12. What is the most common type of brain tumors?
    a. Astrocytoma
    b. Medulloblastoma
    c. Glioblastoma multiforme
    d. Metastatic tumors

13. Radiation treatments that utilize wedges for optimal treatment should be billed as:
    a. Complex simulation
    b. Simple simulation
    c. Complex treatment
    d. Simple treatment

14. Machines with energy ranges of 50-150 kV are known as:
    a. Linear accelerators
    b. Orthovolage
    c. Superficial
    d. Cyclotron

15. Parallel opposed fields have a hinge angle of:
    a. 45 degrees
    b. 90 degrees
    c. 180 degrees
    d. 360 degrees

16. Terrestrial radiation is an example of
    a. Gamma Rays
    b. Natural background radiation
    c. Alpha particles
    d. Beta particles

17. All of the following are environmental factors that can cause nosocomial infections EXCEPT:
    a. Carpeting
    b. Plants
    c. Temperature
    d. Asepsis

18. The gantry, collimator and treatment couch all rotate around the:
    a. Central axis
    b. Target
    c. Isocenter
    d. Past point

19. What is the most common type of skin cancer?
    a. Squamous cell carcinoma
    b. Melanoma
    c. Basal cell carcinoma
    d. Kaposi's sarcoma

20. The portion of the tumor that can be seen or palpated is?
    a. GTV
    b. PTV
    c. ITV
    d. CTV

21. If exposed to radiation during the first 10 days of gestation, what is the most common effect?
    a. Organogenesis
    b. Microcephaly
    c. Skeletal abnormalities
    d. Prenatal death

22. What is true about hand blocks and cast blocks?
    a. Cast blocks are cut to match the angle of the photon beam to reduce penumbra
    b. Hand blocks are custom for each patient
    c. Cast blocks can have 7.5% transmission
    d. A positive block shields the periphery of the radiation field

23. What is the normal range for white blood cells?
    a. 12.0 – 17.5 g/dL
    b. 3.5 – 10.5 billion cells/L
    c. 150,000 – 450,000/mcL
    d. 3.90 – 5.70 million/mcL

24. Which of the following would give the doctor permission to perform a procedure, such as radiation therapy?
    a. Informed Consent
    b. Patient Bill of Rights
    c. Respondeat Superior
    d. Res Ipsa Loquitur

25. What is the d_{max} for a 6 MV beam?
   a. 1.5 cm
   b. 2.5 cm
   c. 3.0 cm
   d. 3.2 cm

26. Which lymph node is located below the mastoid tip and is involved in many head and neck cancers?
   a. Jugulodigastric
   b. Obturator
   c. Mesenteric
   d. Iliac

27. What device is used to spread the beam of electrons when utilizing electron therapy?
   a. Bending magnet
   b. Electron gun
   c. Scattering foil
   d. Flattening filter

28. The distance from the source of radiation to the isocenter is known as:
   a. Source-to-axis distance
   b. Source-to-surface distance
   c. Central axis
   d. Source to collimator distance

29. After what dose would permanent hair loss most likely occur?
   a. 1500 cGy
   b. 2500 cGy
   c. 3500 cGy
   d. 4500 cGy

30. List the following types of radiation in order from LOWEST quality factor to HIGHEST quality factor:
         Alpha particles
         Beta particles
         Neutrons
         Protons
   a. Alpha particles, beta particles, neutrons, protons
   b. Protons, neutrons, beta particles, alpha particles
   c. Beta particles, protons, neutrons, alpha particles
   d. Neutrons, alpha particles, protons, beta particles

31. The Radiation Oncologist wants 100% of the dose to be delivered at the patient's skin surface. The patient is going to be treated with an energy of 6 MV. What bolus thickness would be required?
   a. 0.5 cm
   b. 1.0 cm
   c. 1.5 cm
   d. 2.0 cm

32. The most common pathology for cancers of the oral cavity is:
    a. Adenocarcinoma
    b. Squamous cell carcinoma
    c. Transitional cell carcinoma
    d. Clear cell carcinoma

33. If a patient is not given enough information to make a decision, this type of consent is considered:
    a. Written consent
    b. Verbal consent
    c. Implied consent
    d. Inadequate consent

34. The normal tissue tolerance is 12 Gy and lethal tumor dose is 10 Gy. What is the therapeutic ratio?
    a. 0.8
    b. 1.2
    c. 2.3
    d. 3.6

35. The standard format used to transfer images from diagnostic imaging computers to treatment planning computers is defined by:
    a. DICOM
    b. PACS
    c. DRR
    d. EMR

36. What is the wedge angle needed when there is a hinge angle of 90 degrees?
    a. 15 degrees
    b. 30 degrees
    c. 45 degrees
    d. 60 degrees

37. What can be used to treat anaphylactic shock?
    a. Epinephrine
    b. Methotrexate
    c. Prednisone
    d. Amifostine

38. On a dose-response relationship graph, high LET would be represented as:
    a. A more rounded curve
    b. A slowly declining curve
    c. A steep curve
    d. A flat horizontal line

39. The amount of time the beam is on is known as the:
    a. Occupancy
    b. Dose
    c. Workload
    d. Use factor

40. Tumors that are slow growing and encapsulated are most likely
    a. Superficial
    b. Deep
    c. Benign
    d. Malignant

41. The breast tissue that is located near the axilla is called:
    a. Cooper's ligaments
    b. Tail of Spence
    c. Lattissimus dorsi
    d. Pectoralis minor

42. Which of the following would NOT be included on a radiation therapy treatment prescription?
    a. Beam energy
    b. Dose
    c. Bolus
    d. Monitor units

43. What is the correct order (listed from superior to inferior) of the three divisions of the pharynx?
    a. Oropharynx, nasopharynx, laryngopharynx
    b. Hypopharynx, oropharynx, nasopharynx
    c. Nasopharynx, oropharynx, hypopharynx
    d. Nasopharynx, hypopharynx, oropharynx

44. 1 Gray is equal to how many Sievert?
    a. 1 Sv
    b. 10 Sv
    c. 100 Sv
    d. 1000 Sv

45. If a brain tumor is classified as "well differentiated," it would be given a grade of:
    a. G1
    b. G2
    c. G3
    d. GX

46. What is included in the four "R's" of biologic effectiveness?
    a. Regeneration, redistribution, repair, resolve
    b. Regeneration, repopulation, reoxygenation, repair
    c. Repopulation, redistribution, repair, reoxygenation
    d. Repopulation, regeneration, repair, reoxygenation

47. At what age does the American Cancer Society suggest for men and women to have a screening colonoscopy?
    a. 30
    b. 40
    c. 50
    d. 60

48. What is the equivalent square for a rectangular field measuring 8 cm x 12 cm?
    a. 4.8 cm x 4.8 cm
    b. 9.6 cm x 9.6 cm
    c. 10.5 cm x 10.5 cm
    d. 11.2 cm x 11.2 cm

49. How are tumors accurately diagnosed and staged?
    a. CT simulation
    b. MRI
    c. Mammography
    d. Biopsy

50. The number of waves that pass through a given point in a specified amount of time is known as:
    a. Frequency
    b. Wavelength
    c. Speed
    d. Amplitude

51. Which of the following would be a violation of HIPAA?
    a. Libel
    b. Slander
    c. Negligence
    d. Invasion of Privacy

52. All of the following types of treatment planning require a CT simulator EXCEPT:
    a. 2D
    b. 3D
    c. 4D
    d. IMRT

53. A common chemotherapy drug involved in the treatment of gastrointestinal cancers is:
    a. Methotrexate
    b. Carboplatin
    c. 5 FU
    d. Adriamycin

54. What type of radiation has a charge, heavy mass, high LET and only travels very short distances?
    a. X-rays
    b. Gamma rays
    c. Alpha particles
    d. Beta particles

55. What is the appropriate way to change an error made in the patient's treatment chart?
    a. Cover the error using white out and write the correct entry over it
    b. Draw multiple lines through the error until it is not legible and sign your name
    c. Draw a single line through the error and your initials
    d. Do not make any changes to the error

56. Which of the following is considered an early effect of radiation?
   a. Cataracts
   b. Alopecia
   c. Fibrosis
   d. Leukemia

57. When the treatment room door is opened while the beam is on, the beam should turn off. When the door is shut again what should happen?
   a. The beam should automatically turn on
   b. The patient's treatment cannot be completed
   c. The beam won't turn on until the therapist turns the beam on again
   d. The treatment must start over again

58. What is the type of condition that is associated with cancers of the oral cavity?
   a. Plummer Vinson Syndrome
   b. Familial Adenomatous Polyposis
   c. Ebstein-Barr Virus
   d. Cryptochordism

59. The cause of a disease is defined by:
   a. Epidemiology
   b. Etiology
   c. Screening
   d. Incidence

60. A treatment plan for an AP/PA L-spine requires field weighting. The fields will be weighted 3:1 respectively. If the total dose is 250 cGy, what dose will the AP field receive?
   a. 62.5 cGy
   b. 83.3 cGy
   c. 187.5 cGy
   d. 250.0 cGy

61. What is the most effective way to increase radiation protection?
   a. Decrease time
   b. Increase distance
   c. Increase shielding
   d. Decrease distance

62. At least how much bone marrow needs to be in a treatment field for bone marrow depression to occur?
   a. 10%
   b. 15%
   c. 20%
   d. 25%

63. What is the most common type of soft tissue sarcoma to occur in children?
   a. Ewing sarcoma
   b. Chondrosarcoma
   c. Rhabdomyosarcoma
   d. Malignant fibrous histocytoma

64. IMRT is possible with the use of:
    a. Cerrobend blocks
    b. Compensators
    c. Wedges
    d. MLCs

65. What is the d_{max} for a 9 MeV beam?
    a. 1.5 cm
    b. 2.2 cm
    c. 2.8 cm
    d. 3.0 cm

66. Neutron production can occur in which part of the linear accelerator?
    a. Collimating jaws
    b. Target
    c. Bending magnet
    d. Waveguide

67. Regarding patient billing, "professional" charges are those that involve:
    a. The radiation oncologist
    b. The radiation therapist
    c. The simulation
    d. The treatment

68. A common chemotherapy treatment used to treat Hodgkin's lymphoma is:
    a. CHOP
    b. CMF
    c. MOPP
    d. ABVD

69. All of the following are planes that can be viewed on a CT scan EXCEPT:
    a. Axial
    b. Coronal
    c. Sagittal
    d. Lateral

70. If a person could receive 5 gray in 1 hour within 1 meter from a radiation source, the following sign should be visible:
    a. Radiation area
    b. High radiation area
    c. Very high radiation area
    d. Caution: radioactive materials

71. What is the normal range for platelets?
    a. 12.0 – 17.5 g/dL
    b. 3.5 – 10.5 billion cells/L
    c. 150,000 – 450,000/mcL
    d. 3.90 – 5.70 million/mcL

72. What is the most common type of primary brain tumor in children?
    a. Astrocytoma
    b. Medulloblastoma
    c. Glioblastoma multiforme
    d. Ependymoma

73. The radiation beam has an intensity of 50 mR/hr at a distance of 20 cm from the source. What is the intensity at 12 cm from the source?
    a. 18 mR/hr
    b. 30 mR/hr
    c. 95 mR/hr
    d. 139 mR/hr

74. What is the most sensitive part of the human cell?
    a. RNA
    b. DNA
    c. Proteins
    d. Mitochondria

75. What does "B.I.D." treatment mean?
    a. Two treatments in one week
    b. Two treatments in one day
    c. Three treatments in one week
    d. Three treatments in one day

76. An alpha cradle is what type of immobilization device?
    a. Positioning aid
    b. Simple immobilization device
    c. Complex immobilization device

77. What radiation therapy technique would produce the most accurate positioning for patient treatment?
    a. IGRT
    b. IMRT
    c. Weekly port films
    d. Triangulation

78. All of the following have a quality factor of "1" EXCEPT:
    a. X-rays
    b. Gamma Rays
    c. Beta Particles
    d. Alpha Particles

79. What are the two most toxic materials in Cerrobend blocks?
    a. Tin and Cadmium
    b. Lead and Bismuth
    c. Bismuth and Tin
    d. Cadmium and Lead

80. The klystron is located within the:
    a. Drive stand
    b. Gantry
    c. Collimator
    d. Modulator cabinet

81. What staging system is used for gynecological cancers?
    a. Dukes
    b. Clarks
    c. Ann Arbor
    d. FIGO

82. What is the term that describes the various shades of gray that is present on a CT image?
    a. Window level
    b. Window median
    c. Window width
    d. Window height

83. Where is the most common location for pancreatic tumors to arise?
    a. Body
    b. Tail
    c. Head
    d. Fundus

84. What document defines the patient's expectations of the hospital and gives the patient the right to influence their treatment?
    a. Code of Ethics
    b. Scope of Practice
    c. Patient's Bill of Rights
    d. Health Care Proxy

85. Where is the field size defined?
    a. On the patient's skin surface
    b. At the isocenter
    c. In the collimator
    d. At the source of radiation

86. Characteristic x-rays are a secondary reaction to which photon interaction?
    a. Coherent scattering
    b. Photoelectric effect
    c. Compton scattering
    d. Pair production

87. What does the Pap smear screen for?
    a. Prostate cancer
    b. Cervical cancer
    c. Breast cancer
    d. Rectal cancer

88. Which of the following is NOT a B symptom?
   a. Fever
   b. Night sweats
   c. Hives
   d. Weight loss

89. An orthogonal pair of images is considered images that are taken at angles of _____ degrees from each other.
   a. 10
   b. 45
   c. 90
   d. 180

90. What is the SI unit for absorbed dose?
   a. Rad
   b. Gray
   c. Sievert
   d. Rem

91. The CT number for water is?
   a. -1000
   b. 0
   c. 1
   d. 1000

92. When transferring a patient from a wheelchair to the treatment table, the patient to hold on to the lifter's:
   a. Hands
   b. Arms
   c. Shoulders
   d. Neck

93. The oxygen enhancement ratio describes:
   a. Oxygen enhances survival rates during radiation treatments
   b. Oxygen helps cells repair while radiation is being delivered
   c. Oxygen makes a cell more sensitive to radiation during treatments
   d. Oxygen does not effect radiation treatments

94. Arteriovenous Malformations are most likely treated with:
   a. Electron beam
   b. Brachytherapy
   c. SBRT
   d. SRS

95. The main function of an immobilization device is to?
   a. Make the patient comfortable during treatment
   b. Create a reproducible setup that can be maintained throughout treatment
   c. Prevent the patient from falling
   d. Prevent the patient from talking throughout the treatment

96. Patients experiencing extreme difficulty swallowing from head and neck treatments may require a
_____ to ensure they receive adequate nutrition.
   a. PEG tube
   b. NG tube
   c. PICC line
   d. Catheter

97. Verbal defamation of character is:
   a. Slander
   b. Libel
   c. Negligence
   d. Assault

98. A liposarcoma tumor is what type of tissue?
   a. Fat
   b. Striated muscle
   c. Cartilage
   d. Smooth muscle

99. A brachytherapy applicator that is used to treat cervical cancer is:
   a. Intraluminal
   b. Intracavitary
   c. Interstitial
   d. Intra-arterial

100. "Exposure" can only be defined at energies less than?
   a. 1 MeV
   b. 2 MeV
   c. 3 MeV
   d. 5 MeV

101. Which of the following is a bowel surgery preserves the anal sphincter?
   a. Anterior resection
   b. Abdominoperineal resection
   c. Pancreaticoduodenectomy
   d. Hysterectomy

102. Why are diagnostic CTs not optimal for treatment planning?
   a. Flat couch top
   b. Small bore
   c. Slice thickness cannot be changed
   d. Spacing between slices cannot be changed

103. Where is the most common location to measure a patient's pulse?
   a. Apical artery
   b. Carotid artery
   c. Radial artery
   d. Femoral artery

104. The most common location for bone metastasis of prostate cancer is?
   a. Ribs
   b. Hip
   c. Spine
   d. Shoulder

105. The cells ability to repair itself is represented in which region of the dose-response relationship graph?
   a. D_o
   b. D_q
   c. n
   d. TD 5/5

106. ALARA stands for?
   a. As Little as Reasonably Affordable
   b. As Low as Reasonably Achievable
   c. As Low as Realistically Attainable
   d. As Little as Realistically Achievable

107. A common chemotherapy combination used to treat breast cancer is
   a. CHOP
   b. CMF
   c. MOPP
   d. ABVD

108. Which of the following is primarily used to treat small tumors within the cranium for one fraction using a very high dose?
   a. Intensity-modulated radiation therapy
   b. Total-body irradiation
   c. Stereotactic radiosurgery
   d. Stereotactic body radiation therapy

109. Radiation can cause damage to organs within the body. If the same cell type replaces cells within this organ, what has occurred?
   a. Regeneration
   b. Repair
   c. Necrosis
   d. Reversal

110. If the dose given for a single treatment fraction is different than _____ of the prescription, it is considered a medical event.
   a. 20%
   b. 30%
   c. 40%
   d. 50%

111. CT simulation laser tolerance is?
    a. ± 1 mm
    b. ± 2 mm
    c. ± 1 cm
    d. ± 2 cm

112. The presence of the Reed-Sternberg cell defines which type of cancer?
    a. Hodgkin's lymphoma
    b. Non-Hodgkin's lymphoma
    c. Chronic Myelogenic Leukemia
    d. Acute Myelogenic Leukemia

113. Which of the following energies is the most penetrating?
    a. Cobalt-60
    b. 10 MeV
    c. 6 MV
    d. 10 MV

114. The vagina is located _____ to the bladder and _____ to the rectum.
    a. Anterior, posterior
    b. Posterior, anterior
    c. Medial, lateral
    d. Superior, inferior

115. Patients should be in a room with negative air pressure when they have:
    a. Influenza
    b. Tuberculosis
    c. Pneumonia
    d. Rubella

116. In what order would the following sources be in if you were to list them from shortest half-life to longest half-life?
        Iodine-125
        Cesium-137
        Iridium-192
        Gold-198
    a. Iodine-125, Cesium-137, Iridium-192, Gold-198
    b. Gold-198, Iodine-125, Iridium-192, Cesium-137
    c. Iodine-125, Gold-198, Cesium-137, Iridium-192
    d. Gold-198, Iridium-192, Iodine-125, Cesium-137

117. What is the most common pathology for bladder cancer?
    a. Squamous cell carcinoma
    b. Transitional cell carcinoma
    c. Adenocarcinoma
    d. Clear cell carcinoma

118. What part of the staging system describes the lymph node involvement?
   a. T
   b. N
   c. M
   d. G

119. A microorganism that is the cause of an infectious disease is called
   a. Pathogen
   b. Reservoir
   c. Droplet
   d. Antigen

120. All of the following are related to indirect effects of radiation EXCEPT:
   a. Water
   b. Free radicals
   c. Hydrogen peroxide
   d. Oxygen

121. All of the following are qualities of melanomas EXCEPT?
   a. Asymmetry
   b. Uneven borders
   c. Non-uniform coloring
   d. Diameters smaller than 6mm

122. Cancer screening tests that can detect cancer in early stages is:
   a. Sensitive
   b. Specific
   c. Detailed
   d. Precise

123. To find the area of an irregularly shaped field use:
   a. Clarkson Integration
   b. Equivalent Square
   c. Monte Carlo Computation
   d. Mayneord "F" Factor

124. A "ready pack" film is taped onto the treatment table. The corners of the light field are traced onto the film. An exposure to the film is then made. The markings and the exposed area are compared. What check is this?
   a. Collimator indicator agreement
   b. Light and radiation field agreement
   c. Multileaf collimator performance
   d. Safety light tests

125. Immunosuppressed patients should follow what type of precaution?
   a. Reverse isolation precaution
   b. Contact precaution
   c. Droplet precaution
   d. Airborne precaution

126. How much of the beam is allowed to go through the collimating jaws?
   a. Less than 0.2%
   b. Less than 0.5%
   c. Less than 2%
   d. Less than 5%

127. What would be used to decrease skin sparing?
   a. Wedges
   b. Compensators
   c. Bolus
   d. IMRT

128. A wall that absorbs scatter radiation is known as a:
   a. Primary barrier
   b. Secondary barrier
   c. Tertiary barrier
   d. Scatter barrier

129. Percocet is what type of medication?
   a. Antiemetic
   b. Analgesic
   c. Anti-inflammatory
   d. Antispasmodic

130. What is the most common pathology for esophageal tumors?
   a. Squamous cell carcinoma
   b. Adenocarcinoma
   c. Small cell carcinoma
   d. Clear cell carcinoma

131. Which of the following is not a stage of grieving according to Elisabeth Kubler-Ross:
   a. Denial
   b. Depression
   c. Anger
   d. Annoyance

132. The most radioresistant cycle of cell division is:
   a. G1
   b. G2
   c. M
   d. S

133. The CT number for air is?
   a. -1000
   b. 0
   c. 100
   d. 1000

134. Forward planning is when the:
   a. Planner chooses desired parameters and then the isodose curves are generated
   b. Planner chooses tolerance doses of all tissues in treatment area and then parameters are created
   c. Planner chooses isodose curves and parameters are created
   d. Planner chooses parameters and isodose curves

135. Another term for cell death is
   a. Acentric
   b. Radiolysis
   c. Apoptosis
   d. Carcinogenesis

136. When a wedge is in the path of the radiation beam:
   a. Beam hardening increases
   b. Beam hardening decreases
   c. PDD increases
   d. PDD decreases

137. Which imaging study injects a radioactive material into a patient before imaging?
   a. Nuclear Medicine
   b. Radiography
   c. Magnetic Resonance Imaging
   d. Computed Tomography

138. When viewing a sagittal slice of the male pelvis, the prostate is located _____ to the rectum and _____ to the bladder.
   a. Anterior, posterior
   b. Posterior, anterior
   c. Superior, inferior
   d. Inferior, superior

139. What document defines the patient's expectations of the hospital and gives the patient the right to influence their treatment?
   a. Code of Ethics
   b. Scope of Practice
   c. Patient's Bill of Rights
   d. Health Care Proxy

140. All of the following are localized treatments EXCEPT?
   a. Surgery
   b. External beam radiation therapy
   c. Chemotherapy
   d. Brachytherapy

141. An example of a hormonal agent used to treat breast cancer is?
   a. Doxorubicin
   b. Methotrexate
   c. Cisplatin
   d. Tamoxifen

142. At least what dose is needed to the lens of the eye to cause blindness?
   a. 100 cGy
   b. 500 cGy
   c. 750 cGy
   d. 1000 cGy

143. At least what distance is needed between the compensator and patient's skin surface to maintain skin sparing during photon therapy treatments?
   a. 10 cm
   b. 20 cm
   c. 30 cm
   d. 40 cm

144. The small bowel can be moved out of the treatment field by using a special board and the patient in which position?
   a. Supine
   b. Prone
   c. Right lateral decubitus
   d. Left lateral decubitus

145. Food, water, and medical equipment are examples of which mode of transmission?
   a. Vehicles
   b. Vectors
   c. Droplets
   d. Direct contact

146. A chemotherapy that can cause cardiac toxicity is?
   a. Adriamycin
   b. Bleomycin
   c. Mitomycin
   d. Actinomycin

147. The beam-flattening filter is used for what type of treatments?
   a. Electron
   b. Proton
   c. Photon
   d. Orthovoltage

148. Cryptochordism increases the risk for what type of cancer?
   a. Testicular
   b. Ovarian
   c. Prostate
   d. Penis

149. List the following in order from smallest volume to largest volume

       PTV

       GTV

       CTV

   a. GTV, PTV, CTV

   b. CTV, GTV, PTV

   c. GTV, CTV, PTV

   d. PTV, GTV, CTV

150. Which instrument would be used to find a misplaced source?

   a. Ion chambers

   b. Geiger-Muller detector

   c. Thermoluminescent dosimeter

   d. Diodes

151. All of the following are common locations for metastatic bone disease EXCEPT:

   a. Distal femur

   b. Vertebrae

   c. Pelvic bones

   d. Ribs

152. Chest tubes should be kept at what level?

   a. Above patient's chest?

   b. Same level as patient's chest

   c. Below patient's chest?

   d. 18-24" above chest

153. The type of brachytherapy implant used for endometrial cancers is?

   a. Intracavitary implants

   b. Interstitial implants

   c. Intervascular implants

   d. Interluminal implants

154. On a dose-response relationship graph, the portion of the curve that represents 37% of cell survival is:

   a. D_o

   b. D_q

   c. n

   d. TD 5/5

155. Which type of leukemia has stem cells that contain the Philadelphia chromosome?

   a. ALL

   b. AML

   c. CLL

   d. CML

156. Which isodose curve defines the "useful range" of an electron beam?
    a. 50%
    b. 80%
    c. 90%
    d. 100%

157. The term "assault" means:
    a. Harmfully touching another person
    b. Threatening to harm someone
    c. Verbally insulting someone's character
    d. Writing insulting words about someone's character

158. Viewing images after the patient has been treated is considered?
    a. Registration
    b. Reconstruction
    c. Online review
    d. Offline review

159. Which somatic effect does NOT have a threshold?
    a. Stochastic effects
    b. Non-stochastic effects
    c. Direct effects
    d. Indirect effects

160. The most common pathology for tumors within the endometrium is?
    a. Squamous cell carcinoma
    b. Adenocarcinoma
    c. Clear cell adenocarcinoma
    d. Sarcoma

161. A patient who has mouth sores due to his/her treatment should eat foods that are all of the following EXCEPT:
    a. Soft
    b. Bland
    c. Spicy
    d. Room temperature

162. The DRR is created from?
    a. CT
    b. MRI
    c. X-ray
    d. Port film

163. Two posterior spine fields are required to treat a patient. They are treated with 6 MV and to a depth of 5 cm. One field measures 6 cm x 15 cm at 110 SSD. Another field measures 6 cm x 20 cm at 110 SSD. What is the required gap needed for this treatment?
    a. 0.1 cm
    b. 0.3 cm
    c. 0.8 cm
    d. 1.2 cm

164. What is the maximum cumulative dose limit for a 40-year-old radiation therapist?
    a. 5 rem
    b. 20 rem
    c. 40 rem
    d. 80 rem

165. Who is responsible for filling out the prescription for radiation therapy treatments?
    a. Radiation Therapist
    b. Radiation Oncologist
    c. Radiation Physicist
    d. Radiation Dosimetrist

166. Which of the following is considered a minor reaction to contrast media?
    a. Hypertension
    b. Tachycardia
    c. Vascular shock
    d. Hives

167. What is the method of MLC movement when the MLCs only move when the beam is turned off?
    a. Dynamic
    b. Step and shoot
    c. Sliding window
    d. Classic

168. Where does mesothelioma occur?
    a. Centrally located within the lungs
    b. Periphery of the lungs
    c. Lining of the lungs
    d. In the mediastinum

169. What is the main use of sulfur hexafluoride?
    a. Prevents microwaves from flowing back into the klystron
    b. Prevents linear accelerator from overheating
    c. Prevents arcing within the waveguide
    d. Prevents secondary scattering

170. When a brachytherapy source is placed directly into a tube within the body this is?
    a. Intracavitary implants
    b. Interstitial implants
    c. Intervascular implants
    d. Interluminal implants

171. A patient receiving a dose of 3000 cGy to the upper-abdominal region would need which of the following medications to relieve a common side effect?
    a. Antiemetic
    b. Analgesic
    c. Anti-inflammatory
    d. Anti-diarrheal

172. What type of radiation consists of photons that were naturally produced from a nucleus?
   a. X-rays
   b. Gamma rays
   c. Alpha particles
   d. Beta particles

173. When oxygen is present, the cell is:
   a. Radiosensitive
   b. Radioresistant
   c. The same
   d. Dead

174. A patient is to be treated with 6 MV and a depth of 6 cm. The linear accelerator is calibrated to 100 SAD. The patient has a separation of 26 cm. At midplane, the field size is 12x12cm. The field size on the patient's skin is?
   a. 9.1 x 9.1 cm
   b. 10.4x10.4 cm
   c. 11.3x11.3 cm
   d. 13.8x13.8 cm

175. Influenza can be transmitted through which mode of transmission?
   a. Vehicle-borne
   b. Vector-borne
   c. Airborne
   d. Droplet

176. All of the following are true about non-small cell lung cancer EXCEPT:
   a. Connected with tobacco use
   b. More common in women
   c. Tumors are not centrally located
   d. Better prognosis compared to small cell lung cancer

177. A chemotherapy that can be used as a radiosensitizer is?
   a. Cisplatin
   b. Dexamethasone
   c. Doxorubicin
   d. Vincristine

178. What legal document defines the patient's wishes when they are terminally ill?
   a. Power of attorney
   b. Health care proxy
   c. Living will
   d. DNR

179. The depth where the total dose is delivered is known as?
   a. PDD
   b. TMR
   c. D_{max}
   d. PSF

180. Which of the following is not included when calculating radiation barriers?
a. Occupancy of adjacent rooms
b. Monthly dose
c. Workload
d. Distance

181. What is the name of the largest salivary gland?
a. Submandibular gland
b. Sublingual gland
c. Submantle gland
d. Parotid gland

182. A patient's prescribed total dose is 5400 cGy. The patient is prescribed to receive 180 cGy per fraction for 30 fractions at 100 SSD. What is the total dose the patient would receive if they were accidentally treated at 90 SSD?
a. 4374 cGy
b. 4860 cGy
c. 6000 cGy
d. 6666 cGy

183. What electron interaction occurs near the nucleus and causes the electron to change directions?
a. Characteristic radiation
b. Photonuclear reaction
c. Coherent scattering
d. Bremsstrahlung radiation

184. How much beam is permitted to pass through the collimating jaws?
a. 0.2%
b. 0.5%
c. 2%
d. 5%

185. A patient who is undergoing breast cancer treatments is complaining of a skin reaction after receiving 14 treatments at 180 cGy per fraction. Which option is most likely to be her reaction?
a. Faint erythema
b. Erythema
c. Dry desquamation
d. Moist desquamation

186. What is the ratio of absorbed dose at a depth compared to the absorbed dose at d_{max} known as?
a. Percent depth dose
b. D_{max}
c. Dose equilibrium
d. Tissue-air ratio

187. What is the main location of lymphatic drainage for the right breast?
    a. Left axillary nodes
    b. Right axillary nodes
    c. Left supraclavicular nodes
    d. Right supraclavicular nodes

188. What type of instrument is a "Cutie-Pie"?
    a. Ion chamber
    b. Geiger-Muller detector
    c. Thermoluminescent dosimeter
    d. Diode

189. If you want to adjust the contrast of the CT image, you will be adjusting the:
    a. Window width
    b. Window level
    c. Field of view
    d. Scan field of view

190. To use proper body mechanics when lifting a patient, the radiation therapist should utilize the muscles in his/her:
    a. Arms
    b. Back
    c. Legs
    d. Neck

191. A patient is going to be treated on a linear accelerator using an energy of 6 MV to a depth of 5 cm. The SSD is 91 cm. The TAR is 0.875 and the output is 1.02 cGy/mu. The patient will receive 180 cGy per treatment. How many monitor units must be delivered?
    a. 158 MU
    b. 176 MU
    c. 202 MU
    d. 206 MU

192. Chemotherapy is administration into the spinal canal it is known as:
    a. Intraperitoneal
    b. Intrathecal
    c. Intravenous
    d. Intraarterial

193. What is the limit of radiation per year a restricted area can receive?
    a. 1 rem per year
    b. 5 rem per year
    c. 15 rem per year
    d. 150 rem per year

194. Which scatter factor cannot be directly measured?
    a. Scatter factor
    b. Phantom scatter
    c. Backscatter factor
    d. Peak scatter factor

195. Which mode of transmission is the most common way to spread an infection?
   a. Droplet
   b. Airborne
   c. Direct contact
   d. Vehicle-born

196. What is the most common type of breast cancer?
   a. Infiltrating lobular carcinoma
   b. Infiltrating ductal carcinoma
   c. Lobular carcinoma in situ
   d. Ductal carcinoma in situ

197. A thermoplastic mold that is flexible when in hot water and then can mold around the patient's body is also called:
   a. Alpha cradle
   b. Vac-Lok
   c. Aquaplast
   d. Cerrobend

198. Nosocomial infections are infections that are acquired:
   a. At the patient's home
   b. In the hospital
   c. In a foreign country
   d. For the second time in one month

199. What area of the head and neck region is typically treated with a field size of 6x6 cm due to the lack of nodal involvement?
   a. Pharynx
   b. Larynx
   c. Oral cavity
   d. Parotid Glands

200. Which of the following is an example of sterile technique for medical equipment?
   a. Steam under pressure
   b. Boiling water
   c. Virucides
   d. Germicides

Answer Key Test 1

1. a	53. c	105. b	157. b
2. a	54. c	106. b	158. d
3. a	55. c	107. b	159. a
4. c	56. b	108. c	160. b
5. d	57. c	109. a	161. c
6. d	58. a	110. d	162. a
7. a	59. b	111. b	163. c
8. b	60. c	112. a	164. c
9. a	61. b	113. d	165. b
10. b	62. d	114. b	166. d
11. a	63. c	115. b	167. b
12. d	64. d	116. b	168. c
13. c	65. b	117. b	169. c
14. c	66. a	118. b	170. d
15. c	67. a	119. a	171. a
16. b	68. d	120. d	172. b
17. d	69. d	121. d	173. a
18. c	70. c	122. a	174. b
19. c	71. c	123. a	175. d
20. a	72. a	124. b	176. a
21. d	73. d	125. a	177. c
22. a	74. b	126. b	178. c
23. b	75. b	127. c	179. c
24. a	76. c	128. b	180. b
25. a	77. a	129. b	181. d
26. a	78. d	130. b	182. d
27. c	79. d	131. d	183. d
28. a	80. a	132. d	184. b
29. d	81. d	133. a	185. b
30. c	82. c	134. a	186. a
31. c	83. c	135. c	187. b
32. b	84. c	136. a	188. a
33. d	85. b	137. a	189. a
34. b	86. b	138. a	190. c
35. a	87. b	139. c	191. c
36. c	88. c	140. c	192. b
37. a	89. c	141. d	193. a
38. c	90. b	142. d	194. b
39. c	91. b	143. b	195. c
40. c	92. c	144. b	196. b
41. b	93. c	145. a	197. c
42. d	94. d	146. a	198. b
43. c	95. b	147. c	199. b
44. a	96. a	148. a	200. a
45. a	97. a	149. c	
46. c	98. a	150. b	
47. c	99. b	151. a	
48. b	100. c	152. c	
49. d	101. a	153. a	
50. a	102. b	154. a	
51. d	103. c	155. d	
52. a	104. c	156. a	

Practice Test 2

1. The obturator node is most likely associated with a tumor in which organ?
    a. Breast
    b. Head and neck
    c. Prostate
    d. Pancreas

2. Who is allowed to be in a restricted area within the radiation therapy department?
    a. All hospital workers
    b. Radiation workers
    c. General public
    d. Patient's families

3. All of the following have a direct relationship with PDD, EXCEPT?
    a. Energy
    b. Depth
    c. Field size
    d. SSD

4. A patient who has a skin reaction to radiation therapy should follow all of the following EXCEPT:
    a. Use lotions only as prescribed
    b. Ventilate the area
    c. Wash the area with hot water and soap
    d. Avoid direct sunlight to the area

5. What is another name for small cell lung cancer?
    a. Oat cell
    b. Adenocarcinoma
    c. Transitional cell
    d. Mesothelioma

6. A patient's prescribed total dose is 3000 cGy. The patient was prescribed to receive 300 cGy for 10 fractions at 90 SSD. What is the total dose the patient would receive if they were accidentally treated at 100 SSD?
    a. 2430 cGy
    b. 2700 cGy
    c. 3333 cGy
    d. 3704 cGy

7. What is the d_{max} for a 15 MV beam?
    a. 1.5 cm
    b. 2.5 cm
    c. 3.0 cm
    d. 3.2 cm

8. During the M phase of cell division, radiation will:
    a. Have more of an effect on the cell
    b. Have less of an effect on the cell
    c. Have no effect on the cell
    d. Have the same effect on the cell

9. Radiation treatments that use electrons can be billed as a:
    a. Simple treatment
    b. Intermediate treatment
    c. Complex treatment
    d. Simple simulation

10. Gleason grading is used to grade tumors of which organ?
    a. Bladder
    b. Rectum
    c. Prostate
    d. Vagina

11. If a patient has two different types of treatments at the same time, this is termed?
    a. Adjuvant
    b. Sequential
    c. Substantial
    d. Concurrent

12. The rate that energy is transferred to matter as it travels through it is:
    a. LET
    b. RBE
    c. OER
    d. TLD

13. The CT number for bone is?
    a. -1000
    b. 0
    c. 100
    d. 1000

14. Which blood examination tests the kidney and liver function?
    a. TBI
    b. CBC
    c. BUN
    d. Creatinine

15. Which component of the linear accelerator would only amplify microwaves?
    a. RF driver
    b. Klystron
    c. Magnetron
    d. Waveguide

16. What part of the staging system describes metastatic disease
    a. T
    b. N
    c. M
    d. G

17. A patient uses arm-to-foot straps during a head and neck treatment in order to pull the shoulders out of the way of the treatment field. This immobilization device is considered a:
    a. Positioning aid
    b. Simple immobilization device
    c. Complex immobilization device
    d. Simple treatment

18. Safety check tolerance limits are:
    a. 1 degree
    b. 2 mm
    c. 2%
    d. Functional

19. What is the normal range for hemoglobin?
    a. 12.0 – 17.5 g/dL
    b. 3.5 – 10.5 billion cells/L
    c. 150,000 – 450,000/mcL
    d. 3.90 – 5.70 million/mcL

20. Which gynecological cancer is the most deadly?
    a. Endometrial
    b. Ovarian
    c. Cervical
    d. Vaginal

21. A chemotherapy that can cause pulmonary toxicity is?
    a. Adriamycin
    b. Bleomycin
    c. Mitomycin
    d. Actinomycin

22. What is the most common and economical material used for radiation barriers?
    a. Lead
    b. Tungsten
    c. Aluminum
    d. Concrete

23. If a patient has a superficial skin lesion on his/her forehead, the treatment technique most likely used is:
    a. IMRT
    b. Conformal radiation therapy
    c. SRS
    d. Electron therapy

24. The term used to describe how many people have a specific disease is:
    a. Epidemiology
    b. Etiology
    c. Specificity
    d. Sensitivity

25. The most common location for breast cancer to arise is the:
    a. Upper Outer Quadrant
    b. Upper Inner Quadrant
    c. Lower Outer Quadrant
    d. Lower Inner Quadrant

26. Cancer is an example of which somatic effect?
    a. Stochastic effects
    b. Non-stochastic effects
    c. Direct effects
    d. Indirect effects

27. The radiation beam has an intensity of 100 mR/hr at a distance of 15 cm from the source. What is the intensity at 35 cm from the source?
    a. 18 mR/hr
    b. 42 mR/hr
    c. 234 mR/hr
    d. 544 mR/hr

28. Urine drainage bags should be kept at what level?
    a. Above level of patient's chest
    b. Below level of bladder
    c. Above level of bladder
    d. At the same level of the bladder

29. At approximately what vertebral level is the pancreas located?
    a. T10-T11
    b. T11-T12
    c. T12-L1
    d. L1-L2

30. Which instrument is made up of Lithium Fluoride and can store information for weeks?
    a. Ion chambers
    b. Geiger-Muller detector
    c. Thermoluminescent dosimeter
    d. Optically Stimulated Luminescence

31. After aspiration, what percentage of bone marrow cells must be plasma cells to be diagnosed as multiple myeloma?
    a. 5%
    b. 10%
    c. 15%
    d. 20%

32. If the radiation therapist restrains a patient without the appropriate approval from a physician, this is considered:
   a. Assault
   b. False imprisonment
   c. Negligence
   d. Malpractice

33. A common chemotherapy treatment used to treat non-Hodgkin's lymphoma is:
   a. CHOP
   b. CMF
   c. MOPP
   d. ABVD

34. Which magnet arrangement would create a more confined radiation beam?
   a. 0 degrees
   b. 90 degrees
   c. 180 degrees
   d. 270 degrees

35. A treatment plan for an AP/PA T-spine requires field weighting. The fields will be weighted 2:1 respectively. If the total dose is 300 cGy, what dose will the PA field receive?
   a. 100 cGy
   b. 150 cGy
   c. 200 cGy
   d. 300 cGy

36. Which of the following is an example of aseptic technique for medical equipment?
   a. Bactericides
   b. Steam under pressure
   c. Moist heat
   d. Dry heat

37. The part of the skin that produces pigment is:
   a. Melanocyte
   b. Dermis
   c. Epidermis
   d. Stratum basale

38. Which somatic effect depends on the severity of the radiation dose?
   a. Stochastic effects
   b. Non-stochastic effects
   c. Direct effects
   d. Indirect effects

39. Where is "Point A" located?
   a. 2 cm superior to the cervical os and 2 cm lateral to the endocervical canal
   b. 2 cm superior to the cervical os and 5 cm lateral to the endocervical canal
   c. 2 cm superior to the uterus and 2 cm lateral to the vaginal canal
   d. 2 cm superior to the uterus and 5 cm lateral to the vaginal canal

40. All of the following are types of biopsies EXCEPT:
   a. Fine-needle
   b. Past point
   c. Core needle
   d. Incisional

41. Which imaging study uses high frequency sound waves and images soft tissue in the body?
   a. Nuclear Medicine
   b. Ultrasound
   c. Magnetic Resonance Imaging
   d. Computed Tomography

42. What is the most common type of primary brain tumor in adults?
   a. Astrocytoma
   b. Medulloblastoma
   c. Glioblastoma multiforme
   d. Ependymoma

43. According to the law of Bergonie and Tribondeau, which cells are more sensitive to radiation?
   a. Rapidly dividing cells
   b. Differentiated cells
   c. Mature cells
   d. Malignant cells

44. A patient is receiving arc therapy for 34 treatments. The total dose is 54 Gy, with a daily dose of 180 cGy. The arc will deliver 200 MU. The gantry is moving from 330 to 179 in a clockwise rotation. Calculate the arc speed.
   a. 0.76 MU/degree
   b. 0.96 MU/degree
   c. 1.05 MU/degree
   d. 1.32 MU/degree

45. What is the maximum total dose allowed during gestation?
   a. 0.01 rem
   b. 0.05 rem
   c. 0.1 rem
   d. 0.5 rem

46. Which of the following would be included on a radiation therapy treatment prescription?
   a. Bolus
   b. Monitor units
   c. Treatment position
   d. Immobilization device

47. How many lobes are within the right lung?
   a. 1
   b. 2
   c. 3
   d. 4

48. The most common clinical presentation for endometrial cancer is?
    a. Palpable mass
    b. Pelvic pain
    c. Post menopausal bleeding
    d. Abdominal pain

49. If a patient is getting an HDR treatment, what sign should be hanging on the door?
    a. Radiation area
    b. High radiation area
    c. Very high radiation area
    d. Caution: radioactive materials

50. The type of chemotherapy drug that has a chemical structure similar to that of mustard gas is?
    a. Antimetabolite
    b. Alkylating agent
    c. Antitumor antibiotic
    d. Nitrosoureas

51. What is the wedge angle needed when there is a hinge angle of 150 degrees?
    a. 15 degrees
    b. 30 degrees
    c. 45 degrees
    d. 60 degrees

52. Giving a malnourished patient nutrients through an IV is known as
    a. Percutaneous endoscopic gastrostomy
    b. Myelosuppression
    c. Nasogastric tube
    d. Hyperalimentation

53. Which type of leukemia is most common in pediatrics?
    a. ALL
    b. AML
    c. CLL
    d. CML

54. When radiation attenuates matter, the intensity decreases according to which effect?
    a. Attenuation factor
    b. Inverse square law
    c. Photoelectric effect
    d. Compton scattering

55. Which of the following statements is true?
    a. Bigger field sizes cause more scatter
    b. Bigger field sizes cause less scatter
    c. Field sizes have no effect on scatter

56. If the total dose delivered for the patient's entire treatment is different than _____ of the prescription, it is considered a medical event.
   a. 20%
   b. 30%
   c. 40%
   d. 50%

57. If the treatment planner chooses the tolerance doses for the organs at risk as well as tumor volume and then the treatment computer creates a plan, this is most likely?
   a. Forward planning
   b. Inverse planning
   c. 2D planning
   d. 3D planning

58. Which of the following has the highest quality factor?
   a. X-rays
   b. Neutrons
   c. Heavy particles
   d. Electrons

59. A patient's treatment plan consists of 4 fields. One field is going to receive 45 cGy. The wedge factor is 0.72, the output factor is 0.90 cGy/MU and the TMR is 0.765. How many monitor units will be needed for this field?
   a. 50 MU
   b. 65 MU
   c. 91 MU
   d. 363 MU

60. Malnutrition due to an illness is known as:
   a. Anorexia
   b. Cachexia
   c. Kwashiorkor
   d. Marasmus

61. Alpha particles are chemically similar to?
   a. Carbon
   b. Helium
   c. Nitrogen
   d. Hydrogen

62. What is the d_{max} for a 10 MV beam?
   a. 1.5 cm
   b. 2.5 cm
   c. 3.0 cm
   d. 3.2 cm

63. Which of the following is not a daily check for the linear accelerator?
   a. Door interlock
   b. Beam on light
   c. Emergency switches
   d. Audio-visual monitor system

64. Which lymph node of the head and neck region is difficult to reach during surgery?
   a. Delphian node
   b. Jugulodigastric node
   c. Node of Rouviere
   d. Superior deep jugular node

65. What is used during total body irradiation treatments to increase the skin dose without altering the beam's penetration?
   a. Compensator
   b. Wedge
   c. Block
   d. Beam spoiler

66. What is the appropriate ratio of compressions to breaths during CPR for an adult?
   a. 15:2
   b. 20:2
   c. 30:2
   d. 60:2

67. What staging system is used for lymphoma?
   a. Dukes
   b. Clarks
   c. Ann Arbor
   d. FIGO

68. Which of the following would be prescribed if the patient needs an anti-inflammatory medication?
   a. Torecan
   b. Lomotil
   c. Hydrocortisone
   d. Compazine

69. Lymph nodes located on either side of the sternum and could be included in a treatment for breast cancer is?
   a. Supraclavicular nodes
   b. Internal mammary nodes
   c. Axillary nodes
   d. Mediastinal nodes

70. Which of the following is an example of characteristic of a heavy charged particle?
   a. Changes direction quickly
   b. Large mass
   c. Zig-zag path
   d. Travel further than electrons

71. What type of lung cancer is associated with the use of smoking tobacco and is located in the periphery of the lungs?
    a. Small cell lung cancer
    b. Non-small cell lung cancer
    c. Oat cell lung cancer
    d. Mesothelioma

72. What is the limit of radiation per year an unrestricted area can receive?
    a. 0.1 rem per year
    b. 0.5 rem per year
    c. 1 rem per year
    d. 5 rem per year

73. Which imaging technique can visualize the MLCs and treatment field?
    a. CBCT
    b. MVCT
    c. KV-pair
    d. MV portal image

74. What test screens for breast cancer?
    a. Mammography
    b. Pap smear
    c. Colonoscopy
    d. PSA

75. The treatment plan and the linear accelerator communicate through
    a. R&V system
    b. PACS
    c. DICOM
    d. HIPAA

76. Treatment devices that can be reused for multiple patients each day, such as a pillow or a wing board, can be billed as:
    a. Simple devices
    b. Intermediate devices
    c. Complex devices

77. A total dose of 30 Gy is prescribed over 10 fractions. This treatment would most likely be:
    a. Curative
    b. Keloid
    c. Heteroptropic bone
    d. Palliative

78. Which of the following is NOT a characteristic of electrons?
    a. Charged particles
    b. Indirectly ionizing
    c. Travel in a zig-zag path
    d. Scatter easily

79. In order to bring the beam's d_{max} closer to the skin surface and reduce skin sparing, what must be added to the treatment plan for photon therapy?
 a. Wedge
 b. Compensator
 c. Bolus
 d. Blocks

80. All of the following are examples of early effects of radiation EXCEPT:
 a. Nausea
 b. Fatigue
 c. Telangiectasis
 d. Erythema

81. When creating a treatment plan for IMRT, the type of planning used is most likely:
 a. Forward planning
 b. Inverse planning
 c. 2D planning
 d. 3D planning

82. When all organisms and their spores are destroyed, this is termed:
 a. Asepsis
 b. Sterilization
 c. Cleansing
 d. Anti-bacterial

83. The palatine tonsils are located in the:
 a. Nasopharynx
 b. Oropharynx
 c. Hypopharynx
 d. Larynx

84. What is located within the direction of the radiation beam and checks the output for each treatment?
 a. Ion chamber
 b. Modulator
 c. Electron gun
 d. Klystron

85. What is the method of MLC movement when the MLCs move while the beam is being delivered?
 a. Dynamic
 b. Step and shoot
 c. Static
 d. Classic

86. After how many half-lives can radioactive materials be disposed?
 a. 1
 b. 2
 c. 5
 d. 10

87. List the stages of grieving in order:
    a. Denial, Depression, Annoyance, Acceptance
    b. Bargaining, Denial, Depression, Acceptance
    c. Denial, Anger, Bargaining, Depression, Acceptance
    d. Annoyance, Depression, Bargaining, Acceptance

88. What type of radiation has no charge, is manmade and is created after an interaction near a nucleus?
    a. X-rays
    b. Gamma rays
    c. Alpha particles
    d. Beta particles

89. What is the tolerance dose to 3/3 of the brain according to Emami et al.?
    a. 2300 cGy
    b. 3000 cGy
    c. 4500 cGy
    d. 5000 cGy

90. The most common location for vaginal tumors to arise is the?
    a. Anterior wall
    b. Posterior wall
    c. Inferior medial wall
    d. Superior lateral wall

91. A block that is used to shield the periphery of the treatment field and leaves the central portion open is called:
    a. Hand block
    b. Cast block
    c. Negative block
    d. Positive block

92. When using unsealed ionization chambers to measure radiation, what correction factors are needed?
    a. Dose and Depth
    b. Energy and Size
    c. Temperature and Energy
    d. Temperature and Pressure

93. Esophageal cancers in the upper portion are most likely:
    a. Squamous cell carcinoma
    b. Adenocarcinoma
    c. Small cell carcinoma
    d. Clear cell carcinoma

94. The term "battery" means:
    a. Harmfully touching another person
    b. Threatening to harm someone
    c. Verbally insulting someone's character
    d. Writing insulting words about someone's character

95. Where is the most common location for osteosarcomas?
   a. Proximal femur
   b. Distal femur
   c. Ribs
   d. Distal tibia

96. The shoulder region on a dose-response relationship graph represents
   a. The number of cells available
   b. The cells radiosensitivity
   c. The cells ability to repair itself
   d. The cells radioresistance

97. The Gleason grading system takes scores from how many different locations of the organ?
   a. 1
   b. 2
   c. 4
   d. 6

98. What is the equivalent square for a rectangular field measuring 7.5 cm x 14 cm?
   a. 4.8 cm x 4.8 cm
   b. 6.2 cm x 6.2 cm
   c. 9.8 cm x 9.8 cm
   d. 10.4 cm x 10.4 cm

99. What is the normal range for red blood cells?
   a. 12.0 – 17.5 g/dL
   b. 3.5 – 10.5 billion cells/L
   c. 150,000 – 450,000/mcL
   d. 3.90 – 5.70 million/mcL

100. Which isodose curve defines the "therapeutic range" of an electron beam?
   a. 50%
   b. 80%
   c. 90%
   d. 100%

101. What term describes the radiation beam's penetration ability?
   a. Quality factor
   b. Attenuation factor
   c. Charge
   d. Frequency

102. A patient has a tumor in the central nervous system. This patient experiences symptoms like pain, problems with bowel control and bladder control. In which area of the CNS would this tumor most likely be?
   a. Frontal lobe
   b. Parietal lobe
   c. Occipital lobe
   d. Spinal cord

103. Which of the following defines the standards for patient confidentiality?
    a. HIPAA
    b. OSHA
    c. DICOM
    d. HL7

104. When using an isocentric technique, as the gantry rotates to different angles around the patient's body, what will change?
    a. Source-to-axis distance
    b. Source-to-surface distance
    c. Patient position
    d. Patient support assembly

105. 1 Gray is equal to how many rad?
    a. 1 rad
    b. 10 rad
    c. 100 rad
    d. 1000 rad

106. All of the following are characteristics of collimating jaws in modern day linear accelerators EXCEPT:
    a. Moveable
    b. Asymmetric
    c. Tungsten
    d. Cerrobend

107. What is the minimum number of ways a patient must be identified?
    a. 1
    b. 2
    c. 3
    d. 4

108. A spinal field at 110 SSD uses 320 MU for a treatment. What would the new MU be if the doctor changes the SSD to 100?
    a. 264 MU
    b. 290 MU
    c. 352 MU
    d. 387 MU

109. Which of the following is a radioprotector?
    a. Doxorubicin
    b. Amifostine
    c. Cyclophosphamide
    d. 5-FU

110. How many HVLs are required to block all but 5% of the radiation beam?
    a. 2
    b. 3
    c. 4
    d. 5

111. What is the most efficient way to reduce the spread of infection in the healthcare setting?
    a. Gloves
    b. Gowns
    c. Hand Washing
    d. Protective eyewear

112. What part of the body divides stages 1 and 2 from stages 3 and 4 of Hodgkin's lymphoma
    a. Carina
    b. Umbilicus
    c. Diaphragm
    d. Aorta

113. The amount of time it takes a radioactive source to reach half of its original value is known as:
    a. Half-life
    b. Activity
    c. Intensity
    d. Average life

114. What part of the staging system describes the tumor size
    a. T
    b. N
    c. M
    d. G

115. Which of the following imaging studies does NOT use radiation?
    a. Nuclear Medicine
    b. Radiography
    c. Magnetic Resonance Imaging
    d. Computed Tomography

116. In which plane are CT slices originally obtained?
    a. Axial
    b. Coronal
    c. Sagittal
    d. Lateral

117. What is the most common pathology for tumors within the anus?
    a. Adenocarcioma
    b. Transitional cell carcinoma
    c. Squamous cell carcinoma
    d. Merkel cell

118. When is a human the most sensitive to radiation?
    a. Embryo
    b. Childhood
    c. Adolescence
    d. Adulthood

119. A common combination of chemotherapy drugs used to treat breast cancer is:
    a. CMF
    b. ABVD
    c. MOPP
    d. PLV

120. Informed consent must inform the patient about all of the following EXCEPT:
    a. The procedure and treatment
    b. Risks of having the treatment
    c. Alternative treatment options
    d. Costs of treatments

121. When a brachytherapy source is placed directly into the tumor this is?
    a. Intracavitary implants
    b. Interstitial implants
    c. Intervascular implants
    d. Interluminal implants

122. Which of the following is a radiosensitizer?
    a. Doxorubicin
    b. Ethyol
    c. Sulfhydryls
    d. Amifostine

123. 4D treatment planning incorporates _____ in addition to regular treatment planning.
    a. Involuntary motion
    b. Respiratory motion
    c. Multiple treatment sites
    d. Larger treatment margins

124. Which test screens for prostate cancer?
    a. Prostate specific antigen
    b. Prostate sensitive antigen
    c. Prostate significant an
    d. Prostate specific antitoxin

125. Which of the following will have the most skin sparing?
    a. Therapeutic electron beam
    b. Diagnostic x-rays
    c. Orthovoltage
    d. Megavoltage x-rays

126. Which photon interaction has a threshold energy of 1.022 MeV
    a. Photonuclear reaction
    b. Photoelectric effect
    c. Pair production
    d. Compton scattering

127. A leiomyosarcoma tumor is what type of tissue?
   a. Fat
   b. Striated muscle
   c. Cartilage
   d. Smooth muscle

128. Tuberculosis can be transmitted through which mode of transmission?
   a. Vehicle-borne
   b. Vector-borne
   c. Airborne
   d. Droplet

129. Connective tissue in the breast that provides support is called:
   a. Cooper's ligaments
   b. Tail of Spence
   c. Lattissimus dorsi
   d. Pectoralis minor

130. Radiation can cause damage to organs within the body. If a different cell type replaces cells within this organ, what has occurred?
   a. Regeneration
   b. Repair
   c. Necrosis
   d. Reversal

131. The maximum collimator setting on a linear accelerator is 40x40cm at 100 SAD. What extended distance is needed for a TBI treatment in order to cover a field of 100x100 cm?
   a. 200 cm
   b. 250 cm
   c. 300 cm
   d. 350 cm

132. All of the following are contraindications for using contrast media EXCEPT:
   a. Patients under 50
   b. Patients over 50
   c. Patients with impaired kidney function
   d. Patients who have had reactions to contrast media in the past

133. What is the most effective radiosensitizer?
   a. Nitrogen
   b. Oxygen
   c. Hydrogen
   d. Helium

134. What is the term that describes the average level of shades of gray present on a CT image?
   a. Window level
   b. Window median
   c. Window width
   d. Window height

135. If a wedge is added to a field, what needs to change about the MU?
    a. The MU will decrease
    b. The MU will increase
    c. The MU will remain the same

136. The type of anode used in radiation therapy units is:
    a. Flat
    b. Angled
    c. Rotating
    d. Hooded

137. An immobilization device that is made up of a thick plastic bag with small Styrofoam beams and uses a vacuum to shape the bag is called:
    a. Alpha cradles
    b. Vac-Lok
    c. Aquaplast
    d. Cerrobend

138. Who should sign the patient's chart when entering daily treatments?
    a. The Radiation Oncologist who prescribed dose
    b. The Dosimetrist who planned the treatment
    c. The Radiation Therapists involved in that treatment
    d. The Nurses involved in the patient's care

139. What is the d_{max} for a 12 MeV beam?
    a. 1.5 cm
    b. 2.2 cm
    c. 2.8 cm
    d. 3.0 cm

140. Flies, mosquitos and ticks are examples of which mode of transmission?
    a. Vehicles
    b. Vectors
    c. Droplets
    d. Fomites

141. Which type of leukemia has Auer Rods within the leukemic cells?
    a. ALL
    b. AML
    c. CLL
    d. CML

142. A cyclotron is used for what type of treatment?
    a. External beam radiation therapy
    b. Proton therapy
    c. Electron therapy
    d. Orthovoltage therapy

143. A name for a value that represents a specific shade of gray on the CT image is:
   a. Window width
   b. Window level
   c. CT number
   d. CT density

144. Which of the following is NOT a severe reaction to contrast media?
   a. Anaphylactic shock
   b. Unresponsiveness
   c. Nausea
   d. Pallor

145. A chemotherapy that can be used as a radioprotector is?
   a. Amifostine
   b. Etoposide
   c. Tamoxifen
   d. Leuprolide

146. When radioactive seeds are placed within a prostate, this is considered which type of brachytherapy?
   a. Intraluminal
   b. Intracavitary
   c. Interstitial
   d. Intra-arterial

147. DRRs can be created from the CT scans after a process called:
   a. Registration
   b. Reconstruction
   c. Transmission
   d. Transformation

148. Who is responsible for the filling out the patient's prescription?
   a. Radiation Oncologist
   b. Radiation Physicist
   c. Radiation Therapist
   d. Dosimetrist

149. Where does most of the scatter that contributes to the "scatter factor" occur?
   a. Gantry head
   b. Patient
   c. Wedges
   d. Bolus

150. What is the most common way to measure the radiation output in a linear accelerator?
   a. Ion chambers
   b. Geiger-Muller detector
   c. Thermoluminescent dosimeter
   d. Diodes

151. The legal doctrine that states the employee is liable for themselves when they are negligent is known as:
    a. Respondeat superior
    b. Res ipsa loquitur
    c. Tort
    d. Res ipsa superior

152. Tumors that can grow and spread quickly and are not encapsulated are most likely?
    a. Superficial
    b. Deep
    c. Benign
    d. Malignant

153. How frequently must beam output be checked?
    a. Daily
    b. Monthly
    c. Quarterly
    d. Yearly

154. Which of the following energies would have the shortest wavelength?
    a. 15 MV
    b. 6 MV
    c. 9 MeV
    d. 12 MeV

155. When transferring a patient from a wheelchair to the treatment table, the wheelchair should be positioned:
    a. Parallel to the table
    b. Perpendicular to the table
    c. At a 45 degree angle to the table
    d. Away from the table

156. A belly board is used to:
    a. Keep the patient comfortable
    b. Move organs at risk out of the treatment field
    c. Limit patient motion
    d. Moves bowel into the treatment field

157. Which of the following is a result of a photon interacting with a nucleus?
    a. Bremsstrahlung
    b. Photoelectric effect
    c. Compton scattering
    d. Pair production

158. A benign condition of uncontrolled growth of connective tissue is:
    a. Heterotropic bone
    b. Keloid
    c. Arteriovenous Malformation
    d. Sarcoma

159. Which of the following combinations make up Lipowitz metal (Cerrobend)?
   a. Tin, Lead, Cadmium, Bismuth
   b. Iron, Bismuth, Aluminum, Lead
   c. Bismuth, Aluminum, Lead, Cadmium
   d. Lead, Iron, Cadmium, Tin

160. At what vertebral level does the spinal cord end?
   a. T6-T7
   b. T11-T12
   c. L1-L2
   d. L5-S1

161. The best scenario for a therapeutic ratio is:
   a. The lethal tumor dose is higher than normal tissue tolerance
   b. The lethal tumor dose is equal to normal tissue tolerance
   c. The lethal tumor dose is less than normal tissue tolerance

162. If you want to adjust the brightness of your CT image, you will be adjusting the:
   a. Window width
   b. Window level
   c. Field of view
   d. Scan field of view

163. What is the minimum amount of hours that must pass between B.I.D. treatments?
   a. 1
   b. 2
   c. 4
   d. 6

164. All of the following are located within the oral cavity EXCEPT:
   a. Buccal mucosa
   b. Alveolar ridge
   c. Retromolar trigone
   d. Adenoids

165. What is the annual dose limit for a radiation therapist?
   a. 0.1 rem
   b. 0.5 rem
   c. 1 rem
   d. 5 rem

166. Patients with Tuberculosis should follow what type of precaution?
   a. Reverse isolation precaution
   b. Contact precaution
   c. Droplet precaution
   d. Airborne precaution

167. Negatrons and Positrons are types of:
    a. X-rays
    b. Beta particles
    c. Gamma rays
    d. Alpha particles

168. What is a common free radical that results from indirect effects of radiation?
    a. Hydrogen peroxide
    b. Nitric oxide
    c. Superoxide anion
    d. Hydroxyl

169. What is the type of condition that is associated with Hodgkin's lymphoma?
    a. Plummer Vinson Syndrome
    b. Familial Adenomatous Polyposis
    c. Ebstein-Barr Virus
    d. Human Papillomavirus

170. The part of the body that has the most bone marrow is
    a. Shoulder girdle
    b. Pelvis
    c. Femur
    d. Ribs

171. Images within the therapy department are shared and stored through:
    a. DICOM
    b. PACS
    c. DRR
    d. EMR

172. A health care proxy is someone who:
    a. Makes decisions for the patient when they are not able to
    b. Creates the treatment plan for the patients therapy
    c. Provides religious services to patients
    d. Provides counseling and information to patients and their families

173. The wall that absorbs the useful beam is known as a:
    a. Primary barrier
    b. Secondary barrier
    c. Useful barrier
    d. Scatter barrier

174. Transmission through MLC leaves should be less than?
    a. 0.1%
    b. 0.2%
    c. 1%
    d. 2%

175. Cancer screening tests that can determine a certain type of cancer is:
    a. Sensitive
    b. Specific
    c. Detailed
    d. Precise

176. What is the most common pathology for tumors within the anus?
    a. Adenocarcioma
    b. Transitional cell carcinoma
    c. Squamous cell carcinoma
    d. Epidermoid carcinoma

177. Which of the following sets the standards for handling toxic materials such as Cerrobend?
    a. HIPAA
    b. OSHA
    c. DICOM
    d. HL7

178. When treating a superficial lesion with electron therapy on the lip, what can be used to prevent dose to the gingiva?
    a. Block
    b. Transmission filter
    c. Internal shield
    d. Bolus

179. Which component of the linear accelerator would generate microwaves?
    a. Waveguide
    b. Magnetron
    c. Circulator
    d. Electron gun

180. What is the tolerance limit for the optical distance indicator?
    a. ± 1 mm
    b. ± 2 mm
    c. ± 1 cm
    d. ± 2 cm

181. Which of the following is an example of how a droplet infection can be spread?
    a. Sneeze
    b. Touch
    c. Food
    d. Mosquitos

182. When comparing MV port films prior to the treatment, they are compared with?
    a. CT slices
    b. MRI images
    c. DRRs
    d. X-rays

183. What is the SI unit to describe the amount of radiation a person absorbs?
    a. Sievert
    b. Gray
    c. Rem
    d. Rad

184. When a brachytherapy source is placed directly into a vessel this is?
    a. Intracavitary implants
    b. Interstitial implants
    c. Intervascular implants
    d. Interluminal implants

185. Regarding needle safety, therapists must do all of the following EXCEPT:
    a. Discard the needle in a puncture-resistant container
    b. Use a new needle for each patient
    c. Recap needles after use
    d. Report unwarranted needle sticks

186. What is the largest gland in the body?
    a. Liver
    b. Stomach
    c. Adrenal
    d. Pancreas

187. If the lower third of the esophagus receives a dose of 6500 cGy, what would most likely be the effect?
    a. Perforation
    b. Ulceration
    c. Obstruction
    d. Fistula

188. Viewing images before the patient has been treated and making adjustments if necessary is considered?
    a. CT Simulation
    b. Reconstruction
    c. Online review
    d. Offline review

189. What would prevent microwaves from re-entering the klystron?
    a. Magnetron
    b. Modulator
    c. Waveguide
    d. Circulator

190. All of the following are presentations of inflammatory breast cancer EXCEPT:
    a. Peau d'orange
    b. Breast hardening
    c. Erythema
    d. Palpable mass

191. Written defamation of character is:
    a. Slander
    b. Libel
    c. Negligence
    d. Assault

192. What type of device can help reduce hot spots in a treatment plan with multiple fields or compensate for irregular contours?
    a. Bolus
    b. Wedge
    c. Hand Blocks
    d. Cast Blocks

193. Which acute radiation syndrome would occur after a radiation dose of 5,000 cGy to the entire body?
    a. Cerebrovascular syndrome
    b. Gastrointestinal syndrome
    c. Hematopoietic syndrome
    d. Plummer-Vinson syndrome

194. When determining the monitor units needed to treat fields at extended distances, what is needed for calculation?
    a. Clarkson Integration
    b. Equivalent Square
    c. Monte Carlo Computation
    d. Mayneord "F" factor

195. After a dose of 300 cGy to the testes, sterility is most likely
    a. Permanent
    b. Temporary
    c. No effect
    d. Acute

196. Where is the most common location within the oropharynx for cancers to occur?
    a. Adenoids
    b. Tonsils
    c. Vocal chords
    d. Pyriform sinus

197. Cancer screening tests that can determine a certain type of cancer is:
    a. Sensitive
    b. Specific
    c. Detailed
    d. Precise

198. All of the following could be found on the treatment prescription EXCEPT
    a. Total dose
    b. Fractionated dose
    c. Monitor Units
    d. Bolus

199. During the CT simulation, the mA needs to be increased to create a change in the image quality, this will also lead to:
    a. An increased patient dose
    b. A decreased patient dose
    c. The same patient dose
    d. No patient dose

200. In an emergency situation a patient is unable to give consent for a procedure due to their mental state. Therefore someone else has to make this decision for them. This type of consent is:
    a. Written consent
    b. Verbal consent
    c. Implied consent
    d. Inadequate consent

Answer Key Test 2

1. c	53. a	105. c	157. d
2. b	54. a	106. d	158. b
3. b	55. a	107. b	159. a
4. c	56. a	108. a	160. c
5. a	57. b	109. b	161. c
6. a	58. c	110. d	162. b
7. c	59. c	111. c	163. d
8. a	60. b	112. c	164. d
9. c	61. b	113. a	165. d
10. c	62. b	114. a	166. d
11. d	63. c	115. c	167. b
12. a	64. c	116. a	168. a
13. d	65. d	117. c	169. c
14. c	66. c	118. a	170. b
15. b	67. c	119. a	171. b
16. c	68. c	120. d	172. a
17. b	69. b	121. b	173. a
18. d	70. b	122. a	174. d
19. a	71. b	123. b	175. b
20. b	72. b	124. a	176. c
21. b	73. d	125. d	177. b
22. d	74. a	126. c	178. c
23. d	75. a	127. d	179. b
24. a	76. a	128. c	180. b
25. a	77. d	129. a	181. a
26. a	78. b	130. b	182. c
27. a	79. c	131. b	183. a
28. b	80. c	132. a	184. c
29. d	81. b	133. b	185. c
30. c	82. b	134. a	186. a
31. b	83. b	135. b	187. a
32. b	84. a	136. a	188. c
33. a	85. a	137. b	189. d
34. d	86. d	138. c	190. d
35. a	87. c	139. c	191. b
36. a	88. a	140. b	192. b
37. a	89. c	141. b	193. b
38. b	90. b	142. b	194. d
39. a	91. c	143. c	195. b
40. b	92. d	144. d	196. b
41. b	93. a	145. a	197. b
42. c	94. a	146. c	198. c
43. a	95. b	147. b	199. a
44. b	96. c	148. a	200. c
45. d	97. b	149. a	
46. a	98. c	150. a	
47. c	99. d	151. b	
48. c	100. c	152. d	
49. d	101. a	153. a	
50. b	102. d	154. a	
51. a	103. a	155. a	
52. d	104. b	156. b	

References

AAPM Radiation Therapy Task Group No. 45. AAPM Code of Practice for Radiotherapy Accelerators. College Park, MD.: Published for the American Association of Physicists in Medicine by the American Institute of Physics, 1994. Www.aapm.org. American Association of Physicists in Medicine, 1994. Web. <https://www.aapm.org/pubs/reports/RPT_47.pdf>.

Bentel, Gunilla Carleson. Radiation Therapy Planning. New York: McGraw-Hill, Health Professions Division, 1996. Print.

Bissonnette, Jean-Pierre, Peter A. Balter, Lei Dong, Katja M. Langen, and D. Michael Lovelock. "Quality Assurance for Image-guided Radiation Therapy Utilizing CT-based Technologies: A Report of the AAPM TG-179." Medical Physics 39.4 (2012): 1946-963. Web.

Chao, K.S. Clifford., Carlos A. Perez, and Luther W. Brady. Radiation Oncology Management Decisions. 3rd ed. Philadelphia: Lippincott Williams & Wilkins, a Wolters Kluwer Business, 2011. Print.
"Chemotherapy and Side Effects for Non Hodgkin Lymphoma." Cancer Research UK. Cancer Research UK, 12 Sept. 2014. Web. 05 June 2016. <http://www.cancerresearchuk.org/about-cancer/type/non-hodgkins-lymphoma/treatment/chemotherapy/chemotherapy-and-side-effects-for-non-hodgkins-lymphoma>.

Cunningham, J. R. "Tissue Inhomogeneity Corrections in Photon-Beam Treatment Planning." Progress in Medical Radiation Physics (1982): 103-31. American Association of Physicists in Medicine. Medical Physicists Publishing, Aug. 2004. Web. 5 June 2016. <https://www.aapm.org/pubs/reports/RPT_85.pdf>.

"Diethylstilbestrol (DES) and Cancer." National Cancer Institute. National Cancer Institute, 5 Oct. 2011. Web. 05 June 2016. <http://www.cancer.gov/about-cancer/causes-prevention/risk/hormones/des-fact-sheet>.

Dutta, Pinaki R., MD PHD. "PEG Tube for Head & Neck Cancer Radiation." PEG Tube for Head & Neck Cancer Radiation. OncoLink, 4 Feb. 2008. Web. Jan. 2016. <https://www.oncolink.org/experts/article.cfm?id=2490>.

"Family Cancer Syndromes." American Cancer Society, 19, Apr. 2017, www.cancer.org/cancer/cancer-causes/genetics/family-cancer-syndromes.html.

"How Is Small Intestine Adenocarcinoma Staged?" American Cancer Society. American Cancer Society, 9 Feb. 2016. Web. 30 May 2017.

Iwamoto, Ryan R., et al. Manual for Radiation Oncology Nursing Practice and Education. 4th ed., Oncology Nursing Society, 2012.

Kessler, Marc L., Ph.D, and Kelvin Li, M.S. "Image Fusion For Conformal Radiation Therapy." Www.aapm.org. Department of Radiation Oncology, The University of Michigan, 2001. Web. 2016. <https://aapm.org/meetings/2001AM/pdf/7213-95766.pdf>.

Khan, Faiz M. The Physics of Radiation Therapy. Philadelphia: Lippincott Williams & Wilkins, 2003. Print.

Kole, T. (2017, December 20). Personal interview.

Levy, Leia. Mosby's Radiation Therapy Study Guide and Exam Review. St. Louis, MO: Elsevier Mosby, 2011. Print.

Mayo Clinic Staff. "Brain AVM (arteriovenous Malformation)." Overview–Brain AVM (arteriovenous Malformation)–Mayo Clinic. Mayo Clinic, 29 June 2016. Web. Aug. 2016. <http://www.mayoclinic.org/diseases-conditions/brain-avm/home/ovc-20129992>.

Mayo Clinic Staff. "Complete Blood Count (CBC)." Mayo Clinic, Mayo Foundation for Medical Education and Research. 9 Aug, 2017. www.mayoclinic.org/tests-procedures/complete-blood-count/about/pac-20384919.

"Managing Respiratory Arrest." ACLS Certification Institute, acls.com/free-resources/knowledge-base/respiratory-arrest-airway-management/managing-respiratory-arrest.

McDermott, Patrick N., and Colin G. Orton. The Physics & Technology of Radiation Therapy. Madison: Medical Physics, 2010. Print.

Nath, Ravinder, Peter J. Biggs, Frank J. Bova, C. Clifton Ling, James A. Purdy, Jan Van De Geijn, and Martin S. Weinhous. Medical Physics. 7th ed. Vol. 12. College Park, MD.: Published for the American Association of Physicists in Medicine by the American Institute of Physics, 1994. AAPM Code of Practice for Radiotherapy Accelerators. American Association of Physicists in Medicine, July 1994. Web. 5 June 2016. <https://www.aapm.org/pubs/reports/RPT_47.pdf>.

"National Comprehesive Cancer Network." NCCN Chemotherapy Order Templates, www.nccn.org/professionals/OrderTemplates/Default.aspx.
"NCI Dictionary of Cancer Terms." National Cancer Institute. National Institutes of Health, n.d. Web. 05 June 2016. <http://www.cancer.gov/publications/dictionaries/cancer-terms?cdrid=46487>.

"Proton Therapy." Cancer.Net, 8 Feb. 2017, www.cancer.net/navigating-cancer-care/how-cancer-treated-radiation-therapy/proton-therapy.

Purdy, James, Peter Biggs, Charles Bowers, Edgar Dally, Waiter Downs, and Et. Al. Medical Accelerator Safety Considerations. 4th ed. Vol. 20. New York, NY: Published for the American Association of Physicists in Medicine by the American Institute of Physics, 1996. American Association of Physicists in Medicine. Web.

Task Group #65 Radiation Therapy Committee. "Dose-calculation Algorithms in the Context of Inhomogeneity Corrections for High Energy Photon Beams." Medical Physics 36.10 (2009): 4765-775. Www.aapm.org. American Association of Physicists in Medicine, Aug. 2004. Web. <https://www.aapm.org/pubs/reports/RPT_85.pdf>.

Tolerance of normal tissue to therapeutic irradiationInternational Journal of Radiation Oncology, Biology, Physics; v:21 i:1 p:109-22; 5/15/1991 ElsevierEmami, B; Lyman, J; Brown, A; Coia, L; Goitein, M; Munzenrider, J E; Shank, B; Solin, L J; Wesson, Missn:03603016eissn:1879355Xpmid:2032882doi:10.1016/0360-3016(91)90171-Ycode n:IOBPD3lccn:766434426oclcnum:1865944serissn:03603016sereissn:1879355Xitc:33118243itcp:279970https://www.rightfind.com/vlib/order/orderform.aspx?contentid=33118243

"Understanding Immunotherapy." Www.cancer.net. Cancer.Net, Apr. 2017. Web. 30 May 2017.

United States Nuclear Regulatory Commission. "Report and Notification of a Medical Event." NRC: 10 CFR 35.3045 Report and Notification of a Medical Event. United States Nuclear Regulatory Commission, 02 Dec. 2015. Web. Jan. 2016. <http://www.nrc.gov/reading-rm/doc-collections/cfr/part035/part035-3045.html>.

Vann, Anne Marie., Joan Arazie, and Miles Sutton. Radiation Therapy Essentials: Board Preparation Tool. Augusta, GA: RadOnc Publications, 2010. Print.

Washington, Charles M. Washington, and Dennis T. Leaver. Principles and Practice of Radiation Therapy. St. Louis, MO: Mosby Elsevier, 2010. Print.

"What Is Cancer Immunotherapy?" American Cancer Society. The American Cancer Society Medical and Editorial Content Team, 8 Aug. 2016. Web. 30 May 2017.

Williams, Erica Koch. Patient Care. McGraw-Hill, Health Professions Division, 1999

Made in the USA
Coppell, TX
07 January 2021